ESSENTIAL GYNAECOLOGY

Key Topics for Medical Students and Junior Residents

Dr Essam Abdelhakim

Copyright © 2024 Essam Abdelhakim

All rights reserved

The characters and events portrayed in this book are fictitious. Any similarity to real persons, living or dead, is coincidental and not intended by the author.

No part of this book may be reproduced, or stored in a retrieval system, or transmitted in any form or by any means, electronic, mechanical, photocopying, recording, or otherwise, without express written permission of the publisher.

Cover design by: Art Painter
Library of Congress Control Number: 2018675309
Printed in the United States of America

INTRODUCTION

Welcome to **"Essential Gynecology:** A Comprehensive Guide for Medical Students and Residents".

This Book is crafted to serve as a vital resource for medical students, junior residents, and international medical graduates (IMGs) seeking a thorough understanding of gynecology.

What You Will Find Inside:

1. *Core Topics in Gynecology*: Each chapter is dedicated to a specific aspect of gynecology, covering everything from basic anatomy and physiology to complex conditions such as pelvic pain and urinary incontinence.
2. *Clinical Scenarios:* Real-life case scenarios are included to provide context and application for the theoretical knowledge presented.
3. *Multiple-Choice Questions (MCQs):* To help consolidate your learning and prepare for examinations, this eBook features a selection of MCQs for each topic.

NORMAL MENSTRUAL CYCLE AND DISORDERS

Introduction: *The menstrual cycle is a natural process that occurs in women of reproductive age. It involves the cyclical changes in the ovaries and the endometrium, leading to menstruation if fertilization does not occur. The average menstrual cycle lasts 28 days, with variations between 21 and 35 days considered normal. Understanding the menstrual cycle is essential for diagnosing and managing gynecological disorders.*

Phases Of The Menstrual Cycle:

1. Menstrual Phase (Day 1-5): This is marked by the shedding of the endometrial lining, leading to menstrual bleeding.
2. Follicular Phase (Day 1-13): Under the influence of FSH, multiple ovarian follicles begin to mature, with one dominant follicle eventually ovulating.
3. Ovulation (Day 14): A surge in LH leads to the release of an egg from the dominant follicle.
4. Luteal Phase (Day 15-28): The corpus luteum forms and secretes progesterone, preparing the endometrium for implantation.

Common Disorders:

- *Oligomenorrhea*: Infrequent menstruation, often linked to PCOS or thyroid disorders.
- *Menorrhagia:* Excessive menstrual bleeding, which can result from fibroids or coagulation disorders.
- *Dysmenorrhea:* Painful periods, commonly associated with

endometriosis or pelvic inflammatory disease.

Diagnosis and Management:
- *History and Physical Examination:* Key in diagnosing menstrual disorders.
- *Laboratory Tests:* Hormonal assays, thyroid function tests, and coagulation profiles may be needed.
- Imaging: Ultrasound can help diagnose structural causes like fibroids.

- **Treatment:** Depends on the underlying cause, ranging from hormonal therapies to surgical interventions.
- *Dysmenorrhea:* NSAIDs for pain relief, hormonal contraceptives to reduce menstrual flow.
- *Menorrhagia:* Tranexamic acid, hormonal treatments (e.g., levonorgestrel IUD), or surgical options (e.g., endometrial ablation).
- *Oligomenorrhea/Amenorrhea:* Treatment based on underlying cause, such as hormonal therapy for PCOS or lifestyle changes for hypothalamic amenorrhea

Mcq 1: What Is The Average Length Of A Normal Menstrual Cycle?

- A) 21 days
- B) 28 days
- C) 35 days
- D) 40 days

Answer: B) 28 days

Explanation: The average menstrual cycle length is 28 days, though cycles between 21 and 35 days are considered normal.

Mcq 2: Which Hormone Surge Is Responsible For Ovulation?

- A) Follicle-stimulating hormone (FSH)
- B) Luteinizing hormone (LH)
- C) Estrogen
- D) Progesterone

Answer: B) Luteinizing hormone (LH)

Explanation: The surge in LH is responsible for triggering ovulation, the release of an egg from the dominant follicle.

Clinical Scenario 1: A 25-year-old woman presents with a history of irregular menstrual cycles, occurring every 35-40 days. She complains of heavy bleeding during periods and severe lower abdominal pain. An ultrasound reveals multiple small ovarian cysts.
What is the most likely diagnosis?

Answer: Polycystic Ovary Syndrome (PCOS)

Explanation: The combination of oligomenorrhea, menorrhagia, and ultrasound findings of multiple ovarian cysts is suggestive of PCOS, a common endocrine disorder.

Mcq 3: Which Of The Following Is A Common Cause Of Menorrhagia?

- A) Endometriosis
- B) Polycystic Ovary Syndrome (PCOS)
- C) Fibroids (Uterine Leiomyomas)
- D) Ovarian Cancer

Answer: C) Fibroids (Uterine Leiomyomas)

Explanation: Fibroids are a common cause of heavy menstrual bleeding (menorrhagia) due to their effect on the uterine lining.

Clinical Scenario 2: A 30-year-old woman reports severe dysmenorrhea that started in her early 20s. She describes the pain as cramping and localized to the pelvis, especially during menstruation. A pelvic exam is normal, but the pain persists.
What is the next best step in management?

Answer: Diagnostic laparoscopy to evaluate for endometriosis.

Explanation: Severe dysmenorrhea with a normal pelvic exam can be suggestive of endometriosis, which often requires laparoscopy for definitive diagnosis and treatment.

POLYCYSTIC OVARY SYNDROME (PCOS)

Introduction: *Polycystic Ovary Syndrome (PCOS) is a common endocrine disorder affecting women of reproductive age. It is characterized by hyperandrogenism, ovulatory dysfunction, and polycystic ovaries. PCOS is associated with insulin resistance, obesity, and an increased risk of type 2 diabetes and cardiovascular diseases.*

Clinical Features:

- *Menstrual Irregularities*: Oligomenorrhea or amenorrhea.
- *Hyperandrogenism:* Hirsutism, acne, and alopecia.
- *Polycystic Ovaries:* Multiple small follicles seen on ultrasound.
- *Obesity:* Common but not universal.

Diagnosis:

- **Rotterdam Criteria:**

Requires two of the following three:
1. Oligo- or anovulation.
2. Clinical and/or biochemical signs of hyperandrogenism.
3. Polycystic ovaries on ultrasound.

- Exclusion of Other Disorders: Such as thyroid dysfunction and hyperprolactinemia.

Management:
- *Lifestyle Modifications:* Weight loss and exercise are first-line treatments.
- *Pharmacologic Therapy:*

o   Oral Contraceptives: To regulate menstrual cycles and manage hyperandrogenism.

- o Metformin: For insulin resistance and metabolic symptoms.
- o Anti-androgens: Such as spironolactone for hirsutism.
- *Fertility Treatment:* Clomiphene citrate or letrozole for ovulation induction.

Mcq 1: Which Of The Following Is Not A Common Feature Of Pcos?

- A) Hirsutism
- B) Oligomenorrhea
- C) Hyperthyroidism
- D) Insulin resistance

Answer: C) Hyperthyroidism

Explanation: Hyperthyroidism is not a feature of PCOS. PCOS is characterized by hyperandrogenism, menstrual irregularities, and insulin resistance.

Mcq 2: What Is The First-Line Treatment For Regulating Menstrual Cycles In Women With Pcos?

- A) Metformin
- B) Oral contraceptives
- C) Clomiphene citrate
- D) Spironolactone

Answer: B) Oral contraceptives

Explanation: Oral contraceptives are the first-line treatment for regulating menstrual cycles and managing hyperandrogenism in women with PCOS.

Clinical Scenario 1: A 28-year-old woman with a BMI of 32 presents with irregular menstrual cycles and facial hair growth. Laboratory tests reveal elevated testosterone levels and normal TSH. An ultrasound shows multiple small follicles on both ovaries.

What is the most likely diagnosis?

Answer: Polycystic Ovary Syndrome (PCOS)

Explanation: The combination of menstrual irregularities, hirsutism, obesity, elevated testosterone, and polycystic ovaries is characteristic of PCOS.

Mcq 3: Which Medication Is Commonly Used To Treat Insulin Resistance In Pcos?

- A) Spironolactone
- B) Metformin
- C) Clomiphene citrate
- D) Levothyroxine

Answer: B) Metformin

Explanation: Metformin is commonly used to treat insulin resistance in women with PCOS and can also help with menstrual regularity.

ENDOMETRIOSIS

Introduction: *Endometriosis is a chronic gynecological condition where endometrial-like tissue is found outside the uterus, most commonly on the ovaries, fallopian tubes, and pelvic peritoneum. It is associated with chronic pelvic pain, dysmenorrhea, and infertility.*

Pathophysiology: The exact cause of endometriosis is unknown, but several theories exist, including retrograde menstruation, immune system dysfunction, and genetic predisposition.

Clinical Features:
- Chronic Pelvic Pain: Often worsens during menstruation.
- Dysmenorrhea: Severe menstrual pain.
- Dyspareunia: Painful intercourse.
- Infertility: Up to 50% of women with endometriosis experience difficulty conceiving.

Diagnosis:

- Clinical Suspicion: Based on history and symptoms.
- Imaging: Transvaginal ultrasound may show endometriomas ("chocolate cysts").
- Laparoscopy: The gold standard for diagnosis, allowing direct visualization and biopsy of lesions.

Management:
- *Medical Management:*
o   NSAIDs: For pain relief.
o   Hormonal Therapy: Combined oral contraceptives, GnRH agonists, or progestins to suppress ovulation.
- *Surgical Management:*

o   Laparoscopic Excision: To remove endometriotic lesions.
o   Hysterectomy: For severe cases unresponsive to other treatments, particularly if fertility is no longer desired.

Mcq 1: Which Of The Following Is The Gold Standard For Diagnosing Endometriosis?

- A) MRI
- B) Transvaginal ultrasound
- C) Laparoscopy
- D) Pelvic CT scan

Answer: C) Laparoscopy

Explanation: Laparoscopy is the gold standard for diagnosing endometriosis, as it allows direct visualization and biopsy of endometriotic lesions.

Mcq 2: What Is The Most Common Symptom Of Endometriosis?

- A) Amenorrhea
- B) Chronic pelvic pain
- C) Heavy menstrual bleeding
- D) Urinary incontinence

Answer: B) Chronic pelvic pain

Explanation: Chronic pelvic pain, particularly worsening during menstruation, is the most common symptom of endometriosis.

Clinical Scenario 1: A 32-year-old woman presents with severe dysmenorrhea and chronic pelvic pain. She reports pain during intercourse and difficulty conceiving for the past two years. A pelvic ultrasound shows an ovarian cyst with a homogenous, ground-glass appearance.

What is the most likely diagnosis?

Answer: Endometriosis (Endometrioma)

Explanation: The symptoms of dysmenorrhea, chronic pelvic pain, dyspareunia, and infertility, along with the ultrasound finding of an endometrioma, suggest endometriosis.

Mcq 3: Which Of The Following Treatments Is Most Appropriate For A Woman With Endometriosis Who Desires Future Fertility?

- A) Hysterectomy
- B) Laparoscopic excision of endometriotic lesions
- C) Continuous oral contraceptives
- D) Danazol

Answer: B) Laparoscopic excision of endometriotic lesions

Explanation: Laparoscopic excision is the treatment of choice for women with endometriosis who desire future fertility, as it preserves the reproductive organs while removing endometriotic tissue.

FIBROIDS (UTERINE LEIOMYOMAS)

Introduction: *Uterine fibroids, also known as leiomyomas, are benign smooth muscle tumors of the uterus. They are the most common pelvic tumors in women and can vary in size, number, and location within the uterus. While many fibroids are asymptomatic, they can cause significant morbidity in some women.*

Types Of Fibroids:

- Submucosal: Located just beneath the endometrium.
- Intramural: Found within the uterine wall.
- Subserosal: Located just beneath the uterine serosa.
- Pedunculated: Attached to the uterus by a stalk.

Clinical Features:

- Menorrhagia: Heavy menstrual bleeding.
- Pelvic Pressure or Pain: Due to the size or location of the fibroids.
- Infertility: Submucosal fibroids may interfere with implantation.
- Urinary Symptoms: Frequency or urgency due to pressure on the bladder.

Diagnosis:

- Pelvic Examination: May reveal an enlarged, irregularly shaped uterus.
- *Ultrasound:* The first-line imaging modality for identifying and characterizing fibroids.
- MRI: Used in complex cases to better define the anatomy.

Management:

- Observation: For asymptomatic fibroids.
- *Medical Management:*
o   Hormonal Therapy: To reduce bleeding and shrink fibroids (e.g., GnRH agonists, oral contraceptives).
o   Tranexamic Acid: For menorrhagia.
- *Surgical Management:*
o   Myomectomy: Removal of fibroids while preserving the uterus.
o   Hysterectomy: Definitive treatment, especially for those who have completed childbearing.
o   Uterine Artery Embolization (UAE): Minimally invasive option to shrink fibroids by cutting off their blood supply.

Mcq 1: Which Type Of Fibroid Is Most Likely To Cause Heavy Menstrual Bleeding?

- A) Submucosal
- B) Intramural
- C) Subserosal
- D) Pedunculated

Answer: A) Submucosal

Explanation: Submucosal fibroids are located just beneath the endometrium and are most likely to cause heavy menstrual bleeding (menorrhagia).

Mcq 2: Which Imaging Modality Is First-Line For Diagnosing Uterine Fibroids?

- A) MRI
- B) Pelvic X-ray
- C) CT scan
- D) Ultrasound

Answer: D) Ultrasound

Explanation: Ultrasound is the first-line imaging modality for diagnosing and characterizing uterine fibroids.

Clinical Scenario 1: A 40-year-old woman presents with a history of heavy menstrual bleeding and pelvic pressure. On pelvic examination, the uterus is enlarged and irregular in shape. An ultrasound confirms the presence of multiple intramural fibroids.

What is the best initial management?

Answer: Medical management with hormonal therapy or tranexamic acid.
Explanation: In cases of symptomatic fibroids, initial management often includes medical therapy to control symptoms, such as hormonal therapy or tranexamic acid for heavy menstrual bleeding.

Mcq 3: Which Surgical Procedure Involves The Removal Of Fibroids While Preserving The Uterus?

- A) Hysterectomy
- B) Myomectomy
- C) Endometrial ablation
- D) Uterine artery embolization (UAE)

Answer: B) Myomectomy

Explanation: Myomectomy involves the surgical removal of fibroids while preserving the uterus, making it an option for women who wish to maintain fertility.

ABNORMAL UTERINE BLEEDING (AUB)

Introduction: *Abnormal Uterine Bleeding (AUB) refers to any deviation from normal menstrual patterns, including changes in frequency, duration, or amount of bleeding. It can be caused by a variety of underlying conditions, ranging from hormonal imbalances to structural abnormalities.*

Classification (Figo System):

- **PALM (Structural Causes):**
  - P: Polyps
  - A: Adenomyosis
  - L: Leiomyomas (Fibroids)
  - M: Malignancy and Hyperplasia

- **COEIN (Non-structural Causes):**
  - C: Coagulopathy
  - O: Ovulatory Dysfunction
  - E: Endometrial
  - I: Iatrogenic
  - N: Not Yet Classified

Clinical Features:

- Heavy Menstrual Bleeding (HMB): Excessive menstrual blood loss.
- Intermenstrual Bleeding (IMB): Bleeding between periods.

- Postmenopausal Bleeding: Bleeding after menopause, which warrants investigation for malignancy.

Diagnosis:

- History and Physical Examination: To assess the pattern and severity of bleeding.
- Laboratory Tests: CBC, thyroid function tests, and coagulation profile.
- Imaging: Ultrasound is often used to evaluate structural causes like fibroids or polyps.
- Endometrial Biopsy: Especially important in postmenopausal women or those with risk factors for endometrial cancer.

Management:

- *Medical Management:*

o NSAIDs: For pain and to reduce blood loss.
o Hormonal Therapy: Combined oral contraceptives, progestins, or a levonorgestrel-releasing intrauterine system (LNG-IUS).
o Tranexamic Acid: To reduce menstrual blood loss.

- *Surgical Management:*
o Endometrial Ablation: For those who do not wish to preserve fertility.
o Hysterectomy: In cases of refractory AUB or when malignancy is suspected.

Mcq 1: Which Of The Following Is A Structural Cause Of Abnormal Uterine Bleeding According To The Figo Classification?

- A) Coagulopathy
- B) Ovulatory dysfunction
- C) Polyps

- D) Endometrial

Answer: C) Polyps

Explanation: Polyps are a structural cause of abnormal uterine bleeding according to the FIGO classification system.

Mcq 2: Which Of The Following Is An Appropriate First-Line Treatment For Heavy Menstrual Bleeding In A Woman With No Structural Abnormalities?

- A) Endometrial ablation
- B) Levonorgestrel-releasing intrauterine system (LNG-IUS)
- C) Hysterectomy
- D) Myomectomy

Answer: B) Levonorgestrel-releasing intrauterine system (LNG-IUS)

Explanation: The LNG-IUS is an effective first-line treatment for heavy menstrual bleeding in the absence of structural abnormalities, providing both contraception and reduction of bleeding.

Clinical Scenario 1: A 48-year-old woman presents with heavy, irregular periods over the past year. She has no history of bleeding disorders, and her pelvic ultrasound shows a normal endometrial thickness with no structural abnormalities.

What is the next best step in management?

Answer: Hormonal therapy, such as combined oral contraceptives or a levonorgestrel-releasing intrauterine system (LNG-IUS).

Explanation: In the absence of structural abnormalities,

hormonal therapy is an effective first-line option for managing abnormal uterine bleeding.

Mcq 3: What Is The Most Important Investigation In A Postmenopausal Woman Presenting With Uterine Bleeding?

- A) Pelvic ultrasound
- B) CBC
- C) Endometrial biopsy
- D) Thyroid function tests

Answer: C) Endometrial biopsy

Explanation: Endometrial biopsy is crucial in evaluating postmenopausal bleeding to rule out endometrial cancer or hyperplasia.

AMENORRHEA

Introduction: *Amenorrhea is the absence of menstruation. It is classified as primary when menstruation has never occurred by age 15, and secondary when it occurs after a period of normal menstruation but then ceases for three consecutive cycles or more than six months.*

Causes:

- *Primary Amenorrhea:*
o Gonadal Dysgenesis: Turner syndrome.
o Congenital Anomalies: Mullerian agenesis.
o Hypothalamic or Pituitary Disorders: Kallmann syndrome.

- *Secondary Amenorrhea:*
o Pregnancy: Most common cause.
o Polycystic Ovary Syndrome (PCOS).
o Hypothalamic Amenorrhea: Stress, weight loss, excessive exercise.
o Hyperprolactinemia.

Diagnosis:

- History and Physical Examination: Assess pubertal development, weight changes, and stress.
- Laboratory Tests: Pregnancy test, FSH, LH, TSH, prolactin, and androgen levels.
- Imaging: Pelvic ultrasound, MRI for pituitary lesions.
- Karyotyping: In cases of primary amenorrhea with abnormal physical findings.

Management:

- Treat Underlying Cause: For example, weight restoration for hypothalamic amenorrhea, dopamine agonists for hyperprolactinemia.
- Hormone Replacement Therapy (HRT): For hypoestrogenic states to maintain bone health.
- Counseling: Address psychological impact and future fertility concerns.

Mcq 1: Which Of The Following Is The Most Common Cause Of Secondary Amenorrhea?

- A) Turner syndrome
- B) Polycystic Ovary Syndrome (PCOS)
- C) Pregnancy
- D) Hypothyroidism

Answer: C) Pregnancy

Explanation: Pregnancy is the most common cause of secondary amenorrhea and should be ruled out first in all cases.

Mcq 2: Which Hormone Is Typically Elevated In A Patient With Hyperprolactinemia-Related Amenorrhea?

- A) FSH
- B) LH
- C) Estrogen
- D) Prolactin

Answer: D) Prolactin

Explanation: Elevated prolactin levels are associated with hyperprolactinemia, which can lead to secondary amenorrhea.

Clinical Scenario 1: A 17-year-old girl presents with

primary amenorrhea. She has not developed secondary sexual characteristics and her karyotype reveals 45,X.

What is the most likely diagnosis?

Answer: Turner syndrome

Explanation: The presence of primary amenorrhea, lack of secondary sexual characteristics, and a 45,X karyotype are indicative of Turner syndrome.

Mcq 3: Which Of The Following Is A Common Cause Of Hypothalamic Amenorrhea?

- A) Mullerian agenesis
- B) Obesity
- C) Hyperprolactinemia
- D) Excessive exercise

Answer: D) Excessive exercise

Explanation: Excessive exercise is a common cause of hypothalamic amenorrhea due to the suppression of the hypothalamic-pituitary-ovarian axis.

DYSMENORRHEA

Introduction: *Dysmenorrhea refers to painful menstruation. It can be classified as primary (without underlying pathology) or secondary (due to an identifiable cause such as endometriosis or fibroids).*

Causes:

- *Primary Dysmenorrhea:* Related to prostaglandin release during menstruation, leading to uterine contractions and pain.

- *Secondary Dysmenorrhea:*
o   Endometriosis: Presence of endometrial tissue outside the uterus.
o   Adenomyosis: Endometrial tissue within the uterine muscle.
o   Fibroids: Uterine leiomyomas causing pain due to their location or size.

Clinical Features:

- *Primary Dysmenorrhea:* Cramping pain starting just before or during menstruation, often in adolescents or young women.

- *Secondary Dysmenorrhea:* Pain that may begin earlier in the menstrual cycle and persist longer, often associated with other symptoms like heavy bleeding or dyspareunia.

Diagnosis:

- *History:* Detailed menstrual history to differentiate between primary and secondary dysmenorrhea.
- *Physical Examination:* Pelvic exam to identify structural causes.

- *Imaging:* Ultrasound or MRI to evaluate for endometriosis, fibroids, or adenomyosis.

Management:
- *Primary Dysmenorrhea:*
o   NSAIDs: First-line treatment to reduce prostaglandin levels.
o   Hormonal Contraceptives: To suppress ovulation and reduce menstrual pain.

- *Secondary Dysmenorrhea:* Treatment depends on the underlying cause, such as surgery for endometriosis or fibroids.

Mcq 1: What Is The First-Line Treatment For Primary Dysmenorrhea?

- A) Opioids
- B) NSAIDs
- C) Hormonal therapy
- D) Surgery

Answer: B) NSAIDs

Explanation: NSAIDs are the first-line treatment for primary dysmenorrhea as they reduce prostaglandin production, which is responsible for the pain.

Mcq 2: Which Of The Following Is A Common Cause Of Secondary Dysmenorrhea?

- A) Primary ovarian insufficiency
- B) Endometriosis
- C) Polycystic Ovary Syndrome (PCOS)
- D) Anovulation

Answer: B) Endometriosis

Explanation: Endometriosis is a common cause of secondary

dysmenorrhea, characterized by the presence of endometrial tissue outside the uterus.

Clinical Scenario 1: A 25-year-old woman presents with severe menstrual cramps that started a year ago. The pain begins a few days before her period and lasts throughout menstruation. She also reports dyspareunia.

What is the most likely diagnosis?

Answer: Endometriosis

Explanation: The history of dysmenorrhea that started later in life and is associated with dyspareunia suggests secondary dysmenorrhea, likely due to endometriosis.

Mcq 3: Which Diagnostic Test Is Most Helpful In Evaluating A Patient With Suspected Secondary Dysmenorrhea Due To Adenomyosis?

- A) Pelvic X-ray
- B) Hysteroscopy
- C) Pelvic MRI
- D) Endometrial biopsy

Answer: C) Pelvic MRI

Explanation: Pelvic MRI is the most helpful imaging modality to evaluate adenomyosis, providing detailed images of the uterine wall where the condition occurs.

MENOPAUSE AND HORMONE REPLACEMENT THERAPY (HRT)

Introduction: *Menopause is defined as the permanent cessation of menstruation, occurring after 12 consecutive months without a menstrual period, typically around the age of 50. It marks the end of a woman's reproductive years and is associated with a decline in estrogen and progesterone levels.*

Clinical Features:

- Vasomotor Symptoms: Hot flashes and night sweats.
- Genitourinary Syndrome of Menopause (GSM): Vaginal dryness, atrophy, and dyspareunia.
- Osteoporosis: Increased risk due to decreased bone density.
- Mood Changes: Depression, anxiety, and cognitive changes.

Diagnosis:

- *Clinical Diagnosis:* Based on symptoms and menstrual history.
- FSH Levels: Elevated FSH (>30 mIU/mL) can support the diagnosis but is not always necessary.

Management:

- *Lifestyle Modifications:* Regular exercise, healthy diet, and smoking cessation.
- *Hormone Replacement Therapy (HRT):*
o Indications: Severe vasomotor symptoms, prevention of osteoporosis.
o Contraindications: History of breast cancer, cardiovascular disease, thromboembolic disorders.
o Types: Estrogen alone (for women without a uterus) or

combined estrogen-progestin therapy (for women with an intact uterus).
- Non-Hormonal Options: SSRIs, SNRIs, gabapentin, and clonidine for vasomotor symptoms.
- Calcium and Vitamin D Supplementation: For bone health.

Mcq 1: Which Of The Following Is A Contraindication To Hormone Replacement Therapy (Hrt)?

- A) Osteoporosis
- B) Hot flashes
- C) History of breast cancer
- D) Genitourinary syndrome of menopause (GSM)

Answer: C) History of breast cancer

Explanation: A history of breast cancer is a contraindication to HRT due to the increased risk of cancer recurrence with estrogen therapy.

Mcq 2: What Is The Most Common Symptom Of Menopause?

- A) Osteoporosis
- B) Hot flashes
- C) Vaginal atrophy
- D) Urinary incontinence

Answer: B) Hot flashes

Explanation: Hot flashes are the most common symptom of menopause, affecting up to 75% of women.

Clinical Scenario 1: A 52-year-old woman presents with severe hot flashes and night sweats that are affecting her quality of life.

She has no history of cardiovascular disease or breast cancer.

What is the best initial treatment option?

Answer: Hormone Replacement Therapy (HRT)

Explanation: In a woman without contraindications, HRT is the most effective treatment for severe vasomotor symptoms associated with menopause.

Mcq 3: Which Non-Hormonal Therapy Is Effective For Managing Vasomotor Symptoms In Menopausal Women?

- A) Calcium and Vitamin D
- B) SSRIs
- C) Bisphosphonates
- D) Vaginal lubricants

Answer: B) SSRIs

Explanation: SSRIs, particularly paroxetine, are effective non-hormonal options for managing vasomotor symptoms in menopausal women who cannot take HRT.

OVARIAN CYSTS

Introduction: *Ovarian cysts are fluid-filled sacs within or on the surface of the ovaries. They are common in women of reproductive age and can be functional (related to the menstrual cycle) or pathological.*

Types Of Ovarian Cysts:

- *Functional Cysts:*
o   Follicular Cysts: Form when the follicle fails to rupture during ovulation.
o   Corpus Luteum Cysts: Form when the corpus luteum fails to regress after releasing an egg.

- *Pathological Cysts:*
o   Dermoid Cysts (Mature Cystic Teratomas): Contain tissue such as hair, skin, or teeth.
o   Endometriomas: Associated with endometriosis, contain old blood.
o   Cystadenomas: Benign epithelial tumors, can be serous or mucinous.

Clinical Features:

- Asymptomatic: Many ovarian cysts are asymptomatic and found incidentally.
- Pelvic Pain: May occur if the cyst is large, ruptures, or causes ovarian torsion.
- Menstrual Irregularities: Functional cysts may affect menstrual cycles.
- Pressure Symptoms: Large cysts may cause urinary frequency or constipation.

Diagnosis:
- Pelvic Examination: May reveal a palpable adnexal mass.
- Ultrasound: The imaging modality of choice to characterize cyst size, morphology, and complexity.
- CA-125: Tumor marker that may be elevated in ovarian malignancy, particularly in postmenopausal women with complex cysts.

Management:

- *Expectant Management*: For asymptomatic, simple cysts less than 5 cm in premenopausal women.
- Medical Management: Hormonal contraception to prevent the formation of new functional cysts.

- *Surgical Management:*
o   Cystectomy: For persistent, symptomatic, or complex cysts.
o   Oophorectomy: In cases of suspected malignancy, especially in postmenopausal women.

Mcq 1: Which Of The Following Ovarian Cysts Is Most Commonly Associated With Endometriosis?

- A) Dermoid cyst
- B) Endometrioma
- C) Follicular cyst
- D) Corpus luteum cyst

Answer: B) Endometrioma

Explanation: Endometriomas are ovarian cysts associated with endometriosis and are often filled with old blood, giving them a characteristic "chocolate cyst" appearance.

Mcq 2: A 25-Year-Old Woman Presents With Sudden-Onset Pelvic Pain. Ultrasound Shows A 6 Cm Ovarian Cyst With Free Fluid In The Pelvis. What Is The Most Likely Diagnosis?

- A) Ovarian torsion
- B) Cystadenoma
- C) Cyst rupture
- D) Ectopic pregnancy

Answer: C) Cyst rupture

Explanation: The sudden onset of pain and the presence of free fluid suggest that the ovarian cyst has ruptured.

Clinical Scenario 1: A 32-year-old woman is found to have a 4 cm simple ovarian cyst on routine ultrasound. She is asymptomatic.

What is the best management approach?

Answer: Expectant management with follow-up ultrasound.

Explanation: Asymptomatic, simple ovarian cysts less than 5 cm can be managed expectantly with follow-up ultrasound to ensure resolution.

Mcq 3: Which Type Of Ovarian Cyst Is Most Likely To Contain Hair, Skin, Or Teeth?

- A) Serous cystadenoma
- B) Endometrioma
- C) Dermoid cyst
- D) Follicular cyst

Answer: C) Dermoid cyst

Explanation: Dermoid cysts, also known as mature cystic teratomas, can contain various tissue types, including hair, skin, and teeth.

CERVICAL CANCER SCREENING AND PREVENTION

Introduction: *Cervical cancer is one of the most preventable cancers in women, largely due to effective screening programs and vaccination against human papillomavirus (HPV), the primary cause of cervical cancer.*

Etiology:
• Human Papillomavirus (HPV): The primary cause, particularly high-risk types such as HPV-16 and HPV-18.
• Risk Factors: Multiple sexual partners, early sexual activity, smoking, immunosuppression, and a history of sexually transmitted infections (STIs).

Screening:
• Pap Smear (Papanicolaou Test): Detects precancerous changes in the cervical epithelium (cervical intraepithelial neoplasia or CIN).
• HPV DNA Testing: Identifies high-risk HPV types associated with cervical cancer.

Screening Guidelines:

o   Women aged 21-29: Pap smear every 3 years.
o   Women aged 30-65: Pap smear plus HPV testing every 5 years (preferred) or Pap smear alone every 3 years.
o   Women over 65: Screening can be discontinued if they have had adequate prior screening and are not at high risk.

Prevention:

- HPV Vaccination: Recommended for both girls and boys starting at age 11-12, and up to age 26 for those not previously vaccinated.
- Safe Sexual Practices: Condom use and limiting the number of sexual partners
- Regular Screening: Adherence to recommended screening schedules for early detection of precancerous changes.
- Treatment of Precancerous Lesions: Management of cervical intraepithelial neoplasia (CIN) through procedures like cryotherapy, loop electrosurgical excision procedure (LEEP), or conization to prevent progression to cancer.

Diagnosis Of Cervical Cancer:

- *Colposcopy:* Performed after abnormal Pap smear results to examine the cervix more closely and obtain biopsies.
- *Biopsy*: Histological examination of cervical tissue to confirm the presence and type of cancer.
- *Staging:* Includes imaging studies like MRI, CT scans, and PET scans to determine the extent of cancer spread.

Management:
- **Early Stage (Stage I and II):** May involve surgical options such as hysterectomy (simple or radical) or conization for localized disease.
- **Advanced Stage (Stage III and IV):** Treatment often involves a combination of surgery, radiation therapy, and chemotherapy depending on the extent of disease.
- *Follow-Up:* Regular follow-up after treatment is crucial to monitor for recurrence.

Mcq 1: What Is The Primary Cause Of Cervical Cancer?

- A) Chlamydia trachomatis
- B) Human Papillomavirus (HPV)
- C) Herpes Simplex Virus (HSV)

- D) Cytomegalovirus (CMV)

Answer: B) Human Papillomavirus (HPV)

Explanation: HPV, especially high-risk types such as HPV-16 and HPV-18, is the primary cause of cervical cancer.

Mcq 2: At What Age Is It Recommended To Start Cervical Cancer Screening With Pap Smears?

- A) 18 years
- B) 21 years
- C) 25 years
- D) 30 years

Answer: B) 21 years

Explanation: Cervical cancer screening with Pap smears is recommended to begin at age 21, regardless of sexual history.

Clinical Scenario 1: A 30-year-old woman has a Pap smear result showing atypical squamous cells of undetermined significance (ASC-US).

What is the recommended next step in management?

Answer: Perform HPV testing.

Explanation: In women aged 30-65 with an ASC-US Pap result, HPV testing is recommended to determine if high-risk HPV is present, which may necessitate further evaluation.

Mcq 3: Which Of The Following Vaccines Is Recommended For The Prevention Of Cervical

Cancer?

- A) Hepatitis B vaccine
- B) Influenza vaccine
- C) HPV vaccine
- D) Varicella vaccine

Answer: C) HPV vaccine

Explanation: The HPV vaccine is recommended for the prevention of cervical cancer by protecting against high-risk HPV types.

CONTRACEPTION

Introduction: *Contraception refers to methods used to prevent pregnancy. Various options are available, each with different mechanisms, effectiveness, and side effects.*

Types Of Contraception:

1. **Hormonal Methods:**
o   Combined Oral Contraceptives (COCs): Contain estrogen and progestin, inhibit ovulation, and thicken cervical mucus.
o   Progestin-Only Pills (POPs): Suitable for women who cannot use estrogen.
o   Hormonal Injections: Such as Depo-Provera, provide long-term contraception by inhibiting ovulation.
o   Hormonal Implants: Small rods placed under the skin, releasing progestin for several years.

2. **Barrier Methods:**
o   Condoms: Male and female condoms, also provide protection against STIs.
o   Diaphragms and Cervical Caps: Used with spermicide to block sperm entry into the uterus.

3. **Intrauterine Devices (IUDs):**
o   Copper IUD: Non-hormonal, creates an inflammatory response toxic to sperm.
o   Hormonal IUD: Releases progestin, thickens cervical mucus, and thins the endometrial lining.

4. **Permanent Methods:**
o   Tubal Ligation: Surgical procedure to close or block the fallopian tubes.
o   Vasectomy: Surgical procedure to cut or seal the vas deferens in men.

5. **Emergency Contraception:**
o   Emergency Contraceptive Pills (ECPs): Taken within 72-120 hours after unprotected intercourse to prevent ovulation.
o   Copper IUD: Can also be used as emergency contraception if inserted within 5 days after unprotected intercourse.

Counseling And Choice:

- Patient Preferences: Consider lifestyle, health conditions, and personal preferences.
- Effectiveness: Discuss the efficacy of each method and potential side effects.
- Accessibility: Consider insurance coverage and availability.

Mcq 1: Which Contraceptive Method Is Most Effective In Preventing Pregnancy?

- A) Oral contraceptive pills
- B) Male condoms
- C) Copper IUD
- D) Diaphragm

Answer: C) Copper IUD

Explanation: The copper IUD has a very high efficacy rate in preventing pregnancy, close to 99%.

Mcq 2: Which Contraceptive Method Is Suitable For Women Who Cannot Use Estrogen?

- A) Combined oral contraceptives
- B) Progestin-only pills
- C) Hormonal IUD
- D) Copper IUD

Answer: B) Progestin-only pills

Explanation: Progestin-only pills are suitable for women who cannot use estrogen due to health conditions or contraindications.

Clinical Scenario 1: A 28-year-old woman wants a long-term contraception method that does not require daily attention. **What is the most appropriate option?**

Answer: Hormonal IUD or hormonal implant.

Explanation: Both hormonal IUDs and hormonal implants provide long-term contraception without daily administration.

Mcq 3: Which Emergency Contraception Method Can Be Used Up To 5 Days After Unprotected Intercourse?

- A) Levonorgestrel pill
- B) Ulipristal acetate pill
- C) Copper IUD
- D) Both B and C

Answer: D) Both B and C

Explanation: Both ulipristal acetate pills and the copper IUD can be used up to 5 days after unprotected intercourse as emergency contraception.

INFERTILITY

Introduction: *Infertility is defined as the inability to conceive after one year of regular, unprotected intercourse. It affects both partners and can result from a variety of factors.*

Types Of Infertility:

- *Primary Infertility:* When a couple has never conceived.
- *Secondary Infertility:* When a couple has previously conceived but is unable to conceive again.

Causes Of Infertility:

- **Female Factors:**

o   Ovulatory Disorders: Polycystic ovary syndrome (PCOS), hypothalamic amenorrhea.
o   Tubal Factors: Blocked fallopian tubes due to infections or surgery.
o   Uterine Factors: Fibroids, endometriosis, or congenital anomalies.

- **Male Factors:**

o   Sperm Quality and Quantity: Low sperm count (oligospermia), poor sperm motility (asthenozoospermia), or abnormal sperm morphology (teratozoospermia).
o   Ejaculatory Disorders: Retrograde ejaculation or impotence.

- Combined Factors: Sometimes both partners may have contributing factors.

Evaluation:

- **Female Partner:**

o   History and Physical Examination: Assess menstrual cycles,

past medical history, and physical findings.
o   Laboratory Tests: Hormonal evaluations (FSH, LH, estrogen, progesterone).
o   Imaging: Hysterosalpingography (HSG) to assess the patency of the fallopian tubes.
o   Ultrasound: To check for ovarian cysts, fibroids, or other anomalies.

- **Male Partner:**
o   Semen Analysis: To assess sperm count, motility, and morphology.
o   Physical Examination: To identify anatomical abnormalities.

Management:

- *Lifestyle Changes:* Weight management, smoking cessation, and reduction of alcohol intake.
- *Medical Treatments:*
o   Ovulation Induction: Clomiphene citrate, letrozole for female partners.
o   Hormonal Treatments: For male factor infertility, such as hormone replacement.
- *Surgical Treatments:* Laparoscopy for endometriosis, myomectomy for fibroids.
- *Assisted Reproductive Technologies (ART):*
o   Intrauterine Insemination (IUI): Sperm is placed directly into the uterus.
o   In Vitro Fertilization (IVF): Egg retrieval, fertilization in the lab, and embryo transfer.
o   Intracytoplasmic Sperm Injection (ICSI): Direct injection of sperm into the egg.

Mcq 1: What Is The First-Line Diagnostic Test For Evaluating A Woman With Infertility To Assess The Patency Of The Fallopian Tubes?

- A) Pelvic ultrasound
- B) Hysterosalpingography (HSG)
- C) Laparoscopy
- D) Serum progesterone level

Answer: B) Hysterosalpingography (HSG)

Explanation: HSG is the primary test used to evaluate the patency of the fallopian tubes and can also provide information about uterine abnormalities.

Mcq 2: Which Medication Is Commonly Used To Induce Ovulation In Women With Infertility Due To Anovulation?

- A) Metformin
- B) Clomiphene citrate
- C) GnRH agonists
- D) Progesterone

Answer: B) Clomiphene citrate

Explanation: Clomiphene citrate is the first-line medication used to induce ovulation in women with anovulatory infertility.

Clinical Scenario 1: A 35-year-old woman with a history of irregular menstrual cycles is unable to conceive after 12 months of regular, unprotected intercourse.

What is the most appropriate next step in her evaluation?

Answer: Assess ovulatory function and perform a hysterosalpingography (HSG) to evaluate tubal patency.

Explanation: For a woman with irregular cycles, it is important to assess ovulatory function and check for tubal patency as part of the infertility evaluation.

Mcq 3: What Is The Main Advantage Of In Vitro Fertilization (Ivf) Over Intrauterine Insemination (Iui)?

- A) IVF requires less invasive procedures
- B) IVF does not involve the use of hormones
- C) IVF can bypass issues with tubal factor infertility
- D) IVF is less expensive

Answer: C) IVF can bypass issues with tubal factor infertility

Explanation: IVF can bypass issues with tubal factor infertility by allowing fertilization and embryo development to occur outside the body before transferring embryos to the uterus.

PELVIC INFLAMMATORY DISEASE (PID)

Introduction: *Pelvic Inflammatory Disease (PID) is an infection of the female reproductive organs, including the uterus, fallopian tubes, and ovaries. It is often a complication of sexually transmitted infections (STIs) such as chlamydia or gonorrhea.*

Etiology:
- STIs: Chlamydia trachomatis, Neisseria gonorrhoeae.
- Endogenous Flora: Gardnerella vaginalis, Mycoplasma, Ureaplasma.
- Other Causes: Post-abortion or post-surgical infections.

Clinical Features:

- Abdominal/Pelvic Pain: Often diffuse, but may be localized.
- Vaginal Discharge: May be purulent or abnormal.
- Fever: Commonly present.
- Menstrual Irregularities: Abnormal bleeding or spotting.
- Dyspareunia: Pain during intercourse.

Diagnosis:

- Clinical Examination: Tenderness in the lower abdomen, adnexal tenderness, and cervical motion tenderness.
- Laboratory Tests: Elevated white blood cell count, and possible positive STI tests.
- Imaging: Pelvic ultrasound to rule out abscesses or ectopic pregnancy.
- Laparoscopy: May be used to directly visualize and obtain

cultures if the diagnosis is uncertain.

Management:

- Antibiotics: Broad-spectrum coverage for common pathogens. Empirical therapy may include a combination of doxycycline, azithromycin, and metronidazole.
- Hospitalization: May be necessary for severe cases, or if the patient is pregnant or non-compliant.
- Surgical Intervention: For complications such as tubo-ovarian abscesses or severe infection.

Complications:

- Chronic Pelvic Pain: Due to scarring or chronic infection.
- Infertility: Scarring of the fallopian tubes can lead to infertility.
- Ectopic Pregnancy: Increased risk due to tubal damage.

Mcq 1: Which Of The Following Is A Common Causative Organism Of Pelvic Inflammatory Disease (Pid)?

- A) Streptococcus pneumoniae
- B) Escherichia coli
- C) Chlamydia trachomatis
- D) Mycobacterium tuberculosis

Answer: C) Chlamydia trachomatis

Explanation: Chlamydia trachomatis is a common causative organism of PID, often in conjunction with other STIs.

Mcq 2: Which Clinical Sign Is Most Indicative Of Pid?

- A) Absent bowel sounds
- B) Abdominal guarding
- C) Cervical motion tenderness

- D) Jaundice

Answer: C) Cervical motion tenderness

Explanation: Cervical motion tenderness is a classic sign of PID and is indicative of inflammation of the cervix and surrounding structures.

Clinical Scenario 1: A 25-year-old woman presents with lower abdominal pain, fever, and abnormal vaginal discharge. She is sexually active and reports recent unprotected intercourse.

What is the most appropriate initial management?

Answer: Empirical antibiotic therapy.

Explanation: Given the presentation and risk factors, empirical antibiotic therapy targeting common pathogens associated with PID should be initiated while awaiting culture results.

Mcq 3: What Is A Potential Long-Term Complication Of Untreated Pelvic Inflammatory Disease (Pid)?

- A) Chronic pelvic pain
- B) Acute appendicitis
- C) Chronic migraine
- D) Hyperthyroidism

Answer: A) Chronic pelvic pain

Explanation: Chronic pelvic pain is a potential long-term complication of untreated PID due to scarring and persistent inflammation.

SEXUAL DYSFUNCTION

Introduction: *Sexual dysfunction encompasses a range of issues affecting sexual desire, arousal, and satisfaction. It can impact both men and women and may arise from physical, psychological, or relational factors.*

Types Of Sexual Dysfunction:

1. **Female Sexual Dysfunction:**
o   Sexual Desire Disorder: Reduced or absent sexual desire.
o   Sexual Arousal Disorder: Difficulty achieving or maintaining sexual arousal.
o   Orgasmic Disorder: Difficulty achieving orgasm despite adequate sexual stimulation.
o   Pain Disorders: Pain during intercourse, such as vaginismus or dyspareunia.

2. **Male Sexual Dysfunction:**
o   Erectile Dysfunction: Inability to achieve or maintain an erection sufficient for sexual activity.
o   Premature Ejaculation: Ejaculation occurring sooner than desired, either before or shortly after penetration.
o   Delayed Ejaculation: Difficulty or inability to ejaculate despite adequate sexual stimulation.
o   Low Libido: Reduced sexual desire.

Evaluation:

•   History and Physical Examination: Assess sexual history, relationship factors, and medical conditions.
•   Laboratory Tests: Hormonal evaluations, such as testosterone levels for men or thyroid function tests.

- Psychological Assessment: Evaluate for stress, anxiety, depression, or relationship issues.

Management:
- Medical Treatment: Includes medications such as phosphodiesterase-5 inhibitors (e.g., Viagra) for erectile dysfunction or hormonal therapy for low libido.
- Psychotherapy: For issues related to anxiety, depression, or relationship problems.
- Sex Therapy: To address issues related to sexual technique, communication, and intimacy.
- Lifestyle Changes: Addressing contributing factors such as stress, alcohol use, or weight management.

Mcq 1: Which Class Of Medications Is Commonly Used To Treat Erectile Dysfunction?

- A) Antidepressants
- B) Phosphodiesterase-5 inhibitors
- C) Beta-blockers
- D) Antihistamines

Answer: B) Phosphodiesterase-5 inhibitors

Explanation: Phosphodiesterase-5 inhibitors, such as sildenafil (Viagra), are commonly used to treat erectile dysfunction.

Mcq 2: What Is The Primary Treatment Approach For Premature Ejaculation?

- A) Hormonal therapy
- B) Behavioral techniques and desensitization
- C) Phosphodiesterase-5 inhibitors
- D) Antidepressants

Answer: B) Behavioral techniques and desensitization

Explanation: Behavioral techniques and desensitization strategies are primary treatments for premature ejaculation, although certain antidepressants can also be used off-label.

Clinical Scenario 1: A 40-year-old man reports difficulty achieving and maintaining an erection. He has no significant medical history and is not on any medications.

What is the most appropriate initial management?

Answer: Consider a trial of phosphodiesterase-5 inhibitors and evaluate for underlying psychological factors or lifestyle changes.

Explanation: Phosphodiesterase-5 inhibitors are effective for erectile dysfunction, but a thorough assessment for underlying psychological or lifestyle factors should also be conducted.

Mcq 3: What Is A Common Psychological Factor That Can Contribute To Sexual Dysfunction?

- A) Hypoglycemia
- B) Stress and anxiety
- C) Hyperlipidemia
- D) Hypertension

Answer: B) Stress and anxiety

Explanation: Psychological factors such as stress and anxiety can significantly impact sexual function and contribute to sexual dysfunction.

OVARIAN CANCER

Introduction: *Ovarian cancer is one of the most lethal gynecologic malignancies due to its late presentation. The most common type is epithelial ovarian cancer, but other types include germ cell tumors and stromal tumors.*

Risk Factors:

- Age: Most common in women over 50.
- Family History: BRCA1/BRCA2 mutations increase the risk.
- Nulliparity: Women who have never given birth have a higher risk.
- Endometriosis: Increases the risk of certain types of ovarian cancer.

Clinical Features:
- Asymptomatic in Early Stages: Ovarian cancer often presents late.
- Abdominal Bloating and Distension: Due to ascites or a pelvic mass.
- Early Satiety and Weight Loss: From gastrointestinal involvement.
- Pelvic Pain or Pressure: Due to tumor growth.

Diagnosis:

- Pelvic Examination: May reveal an adnexal mass.
- Transvaginal Ultrasound: First-line imaging for evaluating an adnexal mass.
- CA-125 Blood Test: Elevated in many cases of epithelial

ovarian cancer, but not specific.
- CT Scan: For staging and detecting metastasis.
- Surgical Exploration: Required for definitive diagnosis and staging.

Management:

- Surgery: Cytoreductive surgery (debulking) to remove as much tumor as possible.
- Chemotherapy: Platinum-based chemotherapy (e.g., carboplatin) is the standard treatment.
- Targeted Therapy: PARP inhibitors for BRCA-mutated cancers.
- Follow-Up: Regular CA-125 monitoring and imaging to detect recurrence.

Prognosis:
- Depends on Stage: The prognosis is better when detected early, but most cases are diagnosed at an advanced stage.
- 5-Year Survival Rate: Ranges from 90% in stage I to less than 30% in stage IV.

Mcq 1: Which Of The Following Is A Significant Risk Factor For Developing Ovarian Cancer?

- A) Multiparity
- B) Use of oral contraceptives
- C) BRCA1/BRCA2 mutations
- D) Early menopause

Answer: C) BRCA1/BRCA2 mutations

Explanation: BRCA1/BRCA2 mutations significantly increase the risk of ovarian cancer.

Mcq 2: What Is The Primary Role Of Ca-125 In Ovarian Cancer?

- A) Screening for all women
- B) Staging of ovarian cancer
- C) Monitoring treatment response and detecting recurrence
- D) Diagnosis of early-stage ovarian cancer

Answer: C) Monitoring treatment response and detecting recurrence

Explanation: CA-125 is primarily used to monitor treatment response and detect recurrence in women with known ovarian cancer, rather than for screening or early diagnosis.

Clinical Scenario 1: A 60-year-old woman presents with abdominal bloating, early satiety, and weight loss. Physical examination reveals a pelvic mass.

What is the most appropriate initial diagnostic test?

Answer: Transvaginal ultrasound

Explanation: A transvaginal ultrasound is the first-line imaging test for evaluating a pelvic mass and is crucial for assessing the characteristics of the mass in suspected ovarian cancer.

GESTATIONAL TROPHOBLASTIC DISEASE (GTD)

Introduction: *Gestational Trophoblastic Disease (GTD) encompasses a group of pregnancy-related tumors, including benign conditions like hydatidiform mole (complete or partial) and malignant conditions like choriocarcinoma.*

Types Of Gtd:

- *Complete Hydatidiform Mole*: No fetal tissue, abnormal fertilization with two sperm or one sperm that duplicates.
- *Partial Hydatidiform Mole:* Contains abnormal fetal tissue along with molar tissue, triploid karyotype.
- *Invasive Mole:* Molar tissue invades the myometrium.
- *Choriocarcinoma:* Highly malignant, often metastasizes to the lungs and brain.
- *Placental Site Trophoblastic Tumor (PSTT):* Rare, arises from the placental implantation site.

Clinical Features:

- Vaginal Bleeding: Common presenting symptom.
- Uterine Size Larger Than Dates: Discrepancy between uterine size and gestational age.
- Hyperemesis Gravidarum: Severe nausea and vomiting.
- High hCG Levels: Extremely elevated, leading to symptoms like hyperthyroidism.
- Absent Fetal Heart Tones: In the case of complete mole.

Diagnosis:

- Ultrasound: Snowstorm or cluster of grapes appearance for

complete mole, and abnormal placenta with cystic spaces for partial mole.
• Serum hCG: Elevated levels, much higher than expected for gestational age.
• Histopathology: Confirmatory diagnosis after evacuation of the mole.

Management:
• Suction Curettage: Primary treatment for complete or partial mole.
• Follow-Up: Serial hCG measurements to ensure complete resolution and detect malignancy.
• Chemotherapy: For persistent GTD or choriocarcinoma, usually methotrexate or actinomycin D.
• Hysterectomy: Considered in older women who do not desire future fertility.

Complications:

• Persistent GTD: Occurs in about 15-20% of women after a molar pregnancy.
• Metastasis: Particularly in choriocarcinoma, requiring aggressive treatment.
• Recurrent Molar Pregnancy: Risk increases with a history of prior molar pregnancy.

Mcq 1: Which Of The Following Is A Characteristic Feature Of A Complete Hydatidiform Mole On Ultrasound?

- A) Normal fetal development
- B) Multiple cystic spaces, "snowstorm" appearance
- C) Single cyst with a fetal pole
- D) Placenta previa

Answer: B) Multiple cystic spaces, "snowstorm" appearance

Explanation: The "snowstorm" appearance on ultrasound is characteristic of a complete hydatidiform mole.

Mcq 2: What Is The Primary Treatment For A Complete Hydatidiform Mole?

- A) Chemotherapy
- B) Hysterectomy
- C) Suction curettage
- D) Radiation therapy

Answer: C) Suction curettage

Explanation: Suction curettage is the primary treatment for the evacuation of a complete hydatidiform mole.

Clinical Scenario 1: A 25-year-old woman presents with heavy vaginal bleeding at 12 weeks gestation. Ultrasound reveals a "snowstorm" pattern with no identifiable fetus. Her serum hCG is 200,000 mIU/mL.

What is the most likely diagnosis?

Answer: Complete hydatidiform mole

Explanation: The "snowstorm" pattern on ultrasound and extremely high hCG levels are indicative of a complete hydatidiform mole.

ECTOPIC PREGNANCY

Introduction: *An ectopic pregnancy occurs when a fertilized egg implants outside the uterine cavity, most commonly in the fallopian tube. It is a potentially life-threatening condition if not diagnosed and treated promptly.*

Risk Factors:

- Previous Ectopic Pregnancy
- Tubal Surgery or Infection: Including pelvic inflammatory disease (PID).
- Intrauterine Device (IUD) Use
- Assisted Reproductive Technologies: Such as IVF.
- Smoking

Clinical Features:

- Abdominal Pain: Often unilateral and sharp.
- Vaginal Bleeding: Usually light and irregular.
- Amenorrhea: Missed menstrual period.
- Shoulder Tip Pain: Indicative of diaphragmatic irritation from hemoperitoneum.
- Signs of Shock: Hypotension, tachycardia, and dizziness in the case of rupture.

Diagnosis:

- Transvaginal Ultrasound: First-line imaging, looking for an empty uterus and possible adnexal mass.
- Serum hCG: Levels that plateau or rise abnormally suggest an

ectopic pregnancy.
- Culdocentesis: May be used in emergencies to detect hemoperitoneum.
- Laparoscopy: Definitive diagnosis and treatment.

Management:
- Expectant Management: In select cases where the ectopic pregnancy is small and hCG levels are low.
- Medical Management: Methotrexate for stable patients with unruptured ectopic pregnancies and low hCG levels.

•Surgical Management:

o   Salpingostomy: To preserve the fallopian tube.
o   Salpingectomy: Removal of the affected tube, often used in cases of rupture.

Complications:
- Rupture: Leading to life-threatening intra-abdominal hemorrhage.
- Infertility: Due to damage or loss of the fallopian tube.
- Recurrence: Higher risk of future ectopic pregnancies.

Mcq 1: Which Of The Following Is The Most Common Site Of An Ectopic Pregnancy?

- A) Ovary
- B) Cervix
- C) Fallopian tube
- D) Abdominal cavity

Answer: C) Fallopian tube

Explanation: The fallopian tube is the most common site for ectopic pregnancies, accounting for about 95% of cases.

Mcq 2: Which Of The Following Is A Contraindication For Medical Management Of Ectopic Pregnancy With Methotrexate?

- A) Unruptured ectopic pregnancy
- B) Hemodynamically unstable patient
- C) hCG level < 5,000 mIU/mL
- D) No fetal cardiac activity

Answer: B) Hemodynamically unstable patient

Explanation: Methotrexate is contraindicated in hemodynamically unstable patients, who require immediate surgical intervention.

Clinical Scenario 1: A 32-year-old woman presents with lower abdominal pain and light vaginal bleeding. Her last menstrual period was 6 weeks ago. Ultrasound shows an empty uterus and an adnexal mass. Her serum hCG is 1,500 mIU/mL.

What is the most likely diagnosis?

Answer: Ectopic pregnancy

Explanation: The combination of an empty uterus, adnexal mass, and positive hCG test is highly suggestive of an ectopic pregnancy.

PELVIC ORGAN PROLAPSE (POP)

Introduction: *Pelvic Organ Prolapse (POP) occurs when pelvic organs (uterus, bladder, rectum) descend into or outside the vaginal canal due to weakening of the pelvic floor muscles. It can significantly impact quality of life.*

Etiology:

- Childbirth Trauma: Vaginal deliveries, especially with large babies or prolonged labor.
- Aging: Decreased collagen content and pelvic floor muscle weakening.
- Increased Intra-Abdominal Pressure: Chronic cough, obesity, or heavy lifting.
- Genetic Predisposition: Family history of POP.

Clinical Features:

- Vaginal Bulge: Sensation of a bulge or fullness in the vagina.
- Urinary Symptoms: Incontinence, urgency, or difficulty emptying the bladder.
- Bowel Symptoms: Constipation or incomplete bowel movements.
- Sexual Dysfunction: Discomfort or pain during intercourse.
- Back or Pelvic Pain: Due to the prolapse itself or associated muscle strain.

Diagnosis:

- Physical Examination: Pelvic exam with the patient in the lithotomy position; Valsalva maneuver can be used to demonstrate the extent of prolapse.
- Pelvic Ultrasound or MRI: Occasionally used for assessing the

prolapse.
- Urodynamic Testing: If urinary symptoms are significant.

Management:

- *Conservative Management*:
o Pelvic Floor Muscle Exercises (Kegels): Strengthening the pelvic muscles.
o Pessary: A device inserted into the vagina to support the pelvic organs.

- *Surgical Management*:
o Anterior/Posterior Colporrhaphy: Surgical repair of the vaginal walls.
o Sacrocolpopexy: Suspension of the vaginal vault to the sacrum.
o Hysterectomy: Removal of the uterus may be considered if uterine prolapse is significant.
- *Lifestyle Modifications:* Weight management, treatment of chronic cough, and avoidance of heavy lifting.

Complications:
- Urinary Retention: Due to severe cystocele or prolapse.
- Recurrent Prolapse: Even after surgical repair.
- Infection or Ulceration: Due to the exposure of prolapsed tissue.
- Sexual Dysfunction: Ongoing issues even after treatment.

Mcq 1: Which Of The Following Is The Least Invasive Treatment Option For Pelvic Organ Prolapse?

- A) Pessary
- B) Sacrocolpopexy
- C) Colporrhaphy
- D) Hysterectomy

Answer: A) Pessary

Explanation: A pessary is a non-surgical option that can be used to manage pelvic organ prolapse by providing mechanical support.

Mcq 2: What Is The Primary Risk Factor For The Development Of Pelvic Organ Prolapse?

- A) Nulliparity
- B) Chronic cough
- C) Obesity
- D) Multiparity

Answer: D) Multiparity

Explanation: Multiparity, especially with vaginal deliveries, is the primary risk factor for the development of pelvic organ prolapse due to the trauma to pelvic floor muscles.

Clinical Scenario 1: A 60-year-old woman presents with a sensation of vaginal fullness and difficulty with urination. She has a history of three vaginal deliveries. On examination, a cystocele is noted.

What is the most appropriate initial management?

Answer: The most appropriate initial management would be the use of a pessary, along with pelvic floor exercises.

Explanation: A pessary is a non-invasive option that can provide immediate relief from symptoms, and pelvic floor exercises can help strengthen the supporting muscles.

GESTATIONAL DIABETES MELLITUS (GDM)

Introduction: *Gestational Diabetes Mellitus (GDM) is glucose intolerance that develops during pregnancy and typically resolves postpartum. It is associated with both maternal and fetal complications if not properly managed.*

Etiology:
- Insulin Resistance: Pregnancy hormones, such as human placental lactogen, increase insulin resistance.
- Obesity: Increases the risk of developing GDM.
- Family History: A family history of diabetes increases the risk.
- Advanced Maternal Age: Older women are at higher risk for GDM.

Clinical Features:

- Asymptomatic: Most women with GDM do not have noticeable symptoms.
- Polyuria and Polydipsia: Rarely, excessive thirst and urination may occur.
- Excessive Fetal Growth: Large for gestational age fetus (macrosomia) noted on ultrasound.

Screening and Diagnosis:
- Oral Glucose Tolerance Test (OGTT): Typically performed between 24-28 weeks of gestation. A 75g OGTT is commonly used.
    o Fasting Glucose > 92 mg/dL
    o 1-hour Glucose > 180 mg/dL
    o 2-hour Glucose > 153 mg/dL
- Glycosuria: Not a reliable screening method for GDM.

Management:

- Dietary Modifications: First-line treatment includes a balanced diet with appropriate caloric intake.
- Exercise: Regular physical activity to improve insulin sensitivity.
- Glucose Monitoring: Regular monitoring of blood glucose levels.
- Insulin Therapy: Initiated if blood glucose levels remain elevated despite lifestyle modifications.
- Oral Hypoglycemic Agents: Metformin or glyburide may be considered in some cases, but insulin is preferred.
- Fetal Monitoring: Ultrasound to monitor fetal growth and amniotic fluid levels, non-stress tests in the third trimester.

Complications:

- Maternal: Increased risk of preeclampsia, cesarean delivery, and type 2 diabetes later in life.
- Fetal: Macrosomia, shoulder dystocia, neonatal hypoglycemia, and respiratory distress syndrome.
- Long-Term: Increased risk of obesity and type 2 diabetes in offspring.

Mcq 1: Which Of The Following Is The Most Appropriate Time To Screen For Gestational Diabetes Mellitus (Gdm)?

- A) 12-14 weeks of gestation
- B) 16-18 weeks of gestation
- C) 24-28 weeks of gestation
- D) 32-34 weeks of gestation

Answer: C) 24-28 weeks of gestation

Explanation: Screening for GDM is most appropriately done

between 24-28 weeks of gestation when insulin resistance typically increases.

Mcq 2: What Is The First-Line Management For A Pregnant Woman Diagnosed With Gestational Diabetes Mellitus?

- A) Insulin therapy
- B) Dietary modifications and exercise
- C) Metformin
- D) Immediate delivery

Answer: B) Dietary modifications and exercise

Explanation: The first-line management of GDM includes dietary modifications and exercise to control blood glucose levels.

Clinical Scenario 1: A 30-year-old pregnant woman at 26 weeks of gestation is found to have a fasting glucose level of 100 mg/dL, a 1-hour glucose level of 190 mg/dL, and a 2-hour glucose level of 160 mg/dL during an OGTT.

What is the most likely diagnosis?

Answer: The most likely diagnosis is gestational diabetes mellitus (GDM).

Explanation: The glucose levels meet the criteria for diagnosing GDM during the oral glucose tolerance test.

URINARY INCONTINENCE

Introduction: *Urinary incontinence is the involuntary leakage of urine, affecting women of all ages but more commonly in older women. It can significantly impact quality of life and may be associated with other pelvic floor disorders.*

Types Of Urinary Incontinence:

- *Stress Urinary Incontinence (SUI):* Leakage occurs with increased intra-abdominal pressure, such as during coughing, sneezing, or exercising. It is due to weakness in the pelvic floor muscles or the urethral sphincter.
- *Urge Urinary Incontinence (UUI):* Leakage associated with a sudden, intense urge to urinate, often due to detrusor overactivity.
- *Mixed Urinary Incontinence:* A combination of both stress and urge incontinence.
- *Overflow Incontinence:* Leakage due to overdistention of the bladder, often from bladder outlet obstruction or poor detrusor muscle contractility.

Risk Factors:

- Childbirth: Vaginal delivery, especially with large babies, can damage pelvic floor muscles and nerves.
- Aging: Decreased collagen and muscle tone.
- Obesity: Increased intra-abdominal pressure.
- Menopause: Decreased estrogen levels affect the urethral and vaginal tissues.
- Chronic Cough: From smoking or lung disease, increases pressure on the bladder.

Diagnosis:

- History and Physical Examination: Focus on the type and severity of incontinence, bladder diary, and pelvic exam.
- Urinalysis: To rule out infection.
- Urodynamic Studies: To assess bladder function, especially in complex cases.
- Post-Void Residual Volume: Measured by ultrasound to evaluate incomplete bladder emptying.

Management:
- Lifestyle Modifications: Weight loss, fluid management, and avoiding bladder irritants (e.g., caffeine, alcohol).
- Pelvic Floor Muscle Training (Kegels): First-line therapy for stress incontinence.
- Bladder Training: Timed voiding and urge suppression techniques for urge incontinence.

Medications:

o Anticholinergics (e.g., oxybutynin): For urge incontinence.
o Beta-3 Agonists (e.g., mirabegron): Another option for urge incontinence.
o Topical Estrogens: For postmenopausal women with stress incontinence.

- Surgical Treatment:
o Midurethral Sling Procedure: Commonly used for stress incontinence.
o Bladder Neck Suspension: Another option for stress incontinence.
o Botox Injections: For refractory urge incontinence.
o Sacral Nerve Stimulation: For refractory urge incontinence.

Complications:

- Skin Irritation: Due to constant moisture from urine leakage.
- Urinary Tract Infections (UTIs): From incomplete bladder emptying.
- Emotional Distress: Impact on social life and self-esteem.

Mcq 1: Which Type Of Urinary Incontinence Is Most Commonly Associated With Coughing Or Sneezing?

- A) Urge urinary incontinence
- B) Overflow incontinence
- C) Stress urinary incontinence
- D) Mixed urinary incontinence

Answer: C) Stress urinary incontinence

Explanation: Stress urinary incontinence is characterized by leakage of urine during activities that increase intra-abdominal pressure, such as coughing or sneezing.

Mcq 2: Which Of The Following Is The First-Line Treatment For Stress Urinary Incontinence?

- A) Anticholinergic medications
- B) Bladder training
- C) Midurethral sling surgery
- D) Pelvic floor muscle exercises

Answer: D) Pelvic floor muscle exercises

Explanation: Pelvic floor muscle exercises (Kegels) are the first-line treatment for stress urinary incontinence, helping to strengthen the pelvic floor muscles.

Clinical Scenario 1: A 55-year-old woman presents with a complaint of urine leakage when she exercises and when she coughs or sneezes. She has had three vaginal deliveries and is now postmenopausal.

What is the most likely diagnosis, and what initial management would you recommend?

Answer: The most likely diagnosis is stress urinary incontinence. Initial management should include pelvic floor muscle exercises (Kegels) and possibly a referral for physical therapy.

Explanation: The history of urine leakage with increased intra-abdominal pressure and the patient's obstetric history are consistent with stress urinary incontinence.

SEXUALLY TRANSMITTED INFECTIONS (STIS)

Introduction: *Sexually Transmitted Infections (STIs) are infections that are primarily spread through sexual contact. They can affect various parts of the body, including the genital area, and can lead to serious health complications if untreated.*

Common Stis:

- Chlamydia: Caused by Chlamydia trachomatis, often asymptomatic, but can lead to PID and infertility.
- Gonorrhea: Caused by Neisseria gonorrhoeae, presents with purulent discharge, dysuria, and can also cause PID.
- Syphilis: Caused by Treponema pallidum, presents in stages with primary, secondary, latent, and tertiary symptoms.
- Human Papillomavirus (HPV): Causes genital warts and is associated with cervical cancer.
- Herpes Simplex Virus (HSV): Causes painful genital ulcers and recurs with outbreaks.
- HIV: Causes AIDS, a chronic condition that severely weakens the immune system.
- Trichomoniasis: Caused by Trichomonas vaginalis, leads to frothy, greenish vaginal discharge and itching.
- Bacterial Vaginosis: Often associated with an imbalance of normal vaginal flora, causing a fishy odor and discharge.

Risk Factors:

- Multiple Sexual Partners: Increases the risk of exposure.
- Unprotected Sex: Without the use of condoms.
- History of STIs: Previous infections increase the risk of

recurrence.
- Young Age: Particularly in adolescents and young adults.
- Substance Abuse: Can lead to risky sexual behaviors.

Clinical Features:

- Chlamydia and Gonorrhea: Often asymptomatic, but can cause dysuria, discharge, pelvic pain, and in men, epididymitis.
- Syphilis: Primary stage presents with a painless chancre, secondary with rash, latent with no symptoms, and tertiary with severe systemic involvement.
- HPV: Presents as genital warts; some strains lead to cervical dysplasia and cancer.
- HSV: Painful vesicles or ulcers on the genitals, recurrent episodes.
- Trichomoniasis: Vaginal discharge, itching, and dysuria.

Diagnosis:

- Nucleic Acid Amplification Tests (NAATs): Highly sensitive tests for chlamydia and gonorrhea.
- Serologic Tests: For syphilis (RPR, VDRL), HIV, and HSV.
- Pap Smear and HPV Testing: For cervical dysplasia and HPV infection.
- Microscopy: Wet mount for trichomoniasis, clue cells for bacterial vaginosis.

Management:

- **Antibiotics:**
  o Chlamydia: Azithromycin or doxycycline.
  o Gonorrhea: Ceftriaxone plus azithromycin or doxycycline.
  o Syphilis: Penicillin G.
  o Trichomoniasis: Metronidazole or tinidazole.
- **Antiviral Therapy:**

- o   HSV: Acyclovir, valacyclovir for outbreak and suppression.
- o   HIV: Antiretroviral therapy (ART) for life.
- **Prevention:** Use of condoms, regular STI screenings, vaccination for HPV, and safe sexual practices.
- **Partner Notification** and Treatment: Essential to prevent reinfection and further spread.

Complications:

- Pelvic Inflammatory Disease (PID): Resulting from untreated chlamydia or gonorrhea, leading to chronic pelvic pain, ectopic pregnancy, and infertility.
- Cervical Cancer: Linked to persistent HPV infection.
- Neonatal Infections: Transmission of STIs like HSV, HIV, and syphilis during childbirth.

Mcq 1: Which Of The Following Stis Is Most Commonly Associated With The Development Of Cervical Cancer?

- A) Chlamydia
- B) Syphilis
- C) Gonorrhea
- D) Human Papillomavirus (HPV)

Answer: D) Human Papillomavirus (HPV)

Explanation: HPV, particularly high-risk strains like HPV-16 and HPV-18, is strongly associated with the development of cervical cancer.

Mcq 2: Which Of The Following Is The First-Line

Treatment For Chlamydia?

- A) Acyclovir
- B) Metronidazole
- C) Azithromycin
- D) Ceftriaxone

Answer: C) Azithromycin

Explanation: Azithromycin (or alternatively doxycycline) is the first-line treatment for chlamydia infection.

Clinical Scenario 1: A 24-year-old sexually active woman presents with a 2-week history of vaginal discharge and dysuria. She has a new sexual partner and does not consistently use condoms. On examination, there is mucopurulent cervical discharge, and the cervix bleeds on contact.

What is the most likely diagnosis, and what is the appropriate treatment?

Answer: The most likely diagnosis is chlamydia or gonorrhea cervicitis. The appropriate treatment would be ceftriaxone and azithromycin to cover both infections.

Explanation: The clinical presentation is consistent with cervicitis due to chlamydia or gonorrhea. Dual therapy is recommended to cover both potential pathogens.

VAGINITIS AND VULVOVAGINAL INFECTIONS

Introduction: *Vaginitis refers to inflammation of the vagina that can result in discharge, itching, and pain. Vulvovaginal infections are a common cause of vaginitis and include conditions like bacterial vaginosis, candidiasis, and trichomoniasis.*

Types Of Vaginitis And Infections:

- Bacterial Vaginosis (BV): Caused by an imbalance in the vaginal flora, typically an overgrowth of Gardnerella vaginalis.
- Candidiasis: Fungal infection caused by Candida albicans, leading to yeast infection.
- Trichomoniasis: A sexually transmitted infection caused by Trichomonas vaginalis.
- Atrophic Vaginitis: Common in postmenopausal women due to estrogen deficiency, leading to thinning of the vaginal epithelium.

Risk Factors:

- Antibiotic Use: Disrupts normal vaginal flora, leading to overgrowth of opportunistic pathogens.
- Hormonal Changes: Pregnancy, menopause, and hormonal contraceptives can alter vaginal pH.
- Sexual Activity: Multiple partners or unprotected sex increases the risk of STIs like trichomoniasis.
- Poor Hygiene: Can contribute to bacterial imbalance.
- Immunosuppression: Conditions like diabetes or HIV/AIDS increase susceptibility to infections.

Clinical Features:

- Bacterial Vaginosis: Thin, white or gray discharge with a fishy odor, especially after intercourse.
- Candidiasis: Thick, white, curd-like discharge with itching and burning.
- Trichomoniasis: Frothy, yellow-green discharge with a foul odor, itching, and strawberry cervix on examination.
- Atrophic Vaginitis: Dryness, irritation, and sometimes spotting or pain during intercourse.

Diagnosis:
- Microscopy (Wet Mount): Used to identify clue cells in BV, pseudohyphae in candidiasis, and motile trichomonads in trichomoniasis.
- pH Testing: Elevated pH (>4.5) in BV and trichomoniasis; normal pH in candidiasis.
- Amine Test (Whiff Test): A fishy odor when potassium hydroxide (KOH) is added to the discharge, positive in BV.
- Culture: Can be used for persistent or recurrent infections, especially for candidiasis.

Management:
- Bacterial Vaginosis: Metronidazole or clindamycin, oral or vaginal.
- Candidiasis: Fluconazole orally or topical azoles like clotrimazole.
- Trichomoniasis: Metronidazole or tinidazole, treatment of sexual partners is necessary.
- Atrophic Vaginitis: Topical estrogen therapy, lubricants, and moisturizers.

Complications:
- Recurrent Infections: Especially common in candidiasis and BV.

- Pelvic Inflammatory Disease (PID): BV and trichomoniasis can lead to PID if left untreated.
- Preterm Labor: BV is associated with an increased risk of preterm delivery.
- Sexual Dysfunction: Pain and discomfort during intercourse can impact sexual health.

Mcq 1: Which Of The Following Conditions Is Characterized By A Thick, White, Curd-Like Vaginal Discharge And Intense Itching?

- A) Bacterial Vaginosis
- B) Candidiasis
- C) Trichomoniasis
- D) Atrophic Vaginitis

Answer: B) Candidiasis

Explanation: Candidiasis is characterized by thick, white, curd-like discharge with itching and irritation.

Mcq 2: Which Of The Following Is The Most Appropriate Treatment For Bacterial Vaginosis?

- A) Fluconazole
- B) Metronidazole
- C) Clotrimazole
- D) Tinidazole

Answer: B) Metronidazole

Explanation: Metronidazole is the first-line treatment for bacterial vaginosis, available in oral and vaginal formulations.

Clinical Scenario 1: A 30-year-old woman presents with complaints of a fishy-smelling vaginal discharge that worsens after intercourse. She denies itching or pain. On examination, there is a thin, grayish discharge. The pH of the vaginal fluid is 5.5.

What is the most likely diagnosis, and what is the treatment?

Answer: The most likely diagnosis is bacterial vaginosis. The treatment would be metronidazole or clindamycin.
Explanation: The fishy odor, discharge characteristics, and elevated vaginal pH are typical findings in bacterial vaginosis.

PELVIC PAIN

Introduction: *Pelvic pain is a common complaint in women and can be acute or chronic. It may arise from gynecological, urological, gastrointestinal, or musculoskeletal causes. A thorough evaluation is essential to identify the underlying cause and provide appropriate treatment.*

Types Of Pelvic Pain:

- *Acute Pelvic Pain:* Sudden onset, often severe, and may require urgent evaluation. Common causes include ectopic pregnancy, ovarian torsion, and acute pelvic inflammatory disease (PID).
- *Chronic Pelvic Pain:* Persistent pain lasting more than six months, often multifactorial. Conditions include endometriosis, interstitial cystitis, and adhesions.

Common Causes:

- **Gynecological:**
  - Endometriosis: Presence of endometrial tissue outside the uterus causing cyclic pain.
  - Ovarian Cysts: Especially when ruptured or causing torsion.
  - Pelvic Inflammatory Disease (PID): Infection of the upper genital tract, often due to untreated STIs.
  - Fibroids: Non-cancerous tumors of the uterus causing pressure and pain.

- **Urological:**
  - Interstitial Cystitis: Chronic bladder pain syndrome with urgency and frequency.
  - Urinary Tract Infection (UTI): Lower abdominal pain with dysuria.

- **Gastrointestinal:**
o Irritable Bowel Syndrome (IBS): Abdominal pain related to bowel movements.
o Appendicitis: Right lower quadrant pain, often acute.

- **Musculoskeletal:**
o Pelvic Floor Dysfunction: Spasm or weakness of the pelvic floor muscles leading to pain.

Clinical Features:

- Endometriosis: Cyclic pelvic pain, dysmenorrhea, and dyspareunia.
- Ovarian Torsion: Sudden, severe unilateral pain with nausea and vomiting.
- PID: Lower abdominal pain, fever, and cervical motion tenderness.
- Interstitial Cystitis: Chronic pelvic pain, urinary urgency, and frequency without infection.

Diagnosis:

- History and Physical Examination: Focused on the location, duration, and nature of the pain.
- Pelvic Ultrasound: First-line imaging for gynecological causes like ovarian cysts or fibroids.
- Laparoscopy: Definitive for diagnosing endometriosis or chronic pelvic pain of unclear etiology.
- Urinalysis: To rule out UTI.
- STI Screening: For PID, particularly chlamydia and gonorrhea.
- MRI or CT Scan: May be needed for complex cases or to rule out non-gynecological causes.

Management:

- **Medical Treatment:**
o NSAIDs: First-line for pain management.
o Hormonal Therapy: Oral contraceptives, GnRH analogs for endometriosis.
o Antibiotics: For PID or UTI.
o Neuromodulators: For chronic pelvic pain syndromes like interstitial cystitis.

- **Surgical Treatment:**
o Laparoscopy: For diagnosis and treatment of endometriosis, ovarian cysts, or adhesions.
o Hysterectomy: In cases of severe pain from fibroids or endometriosis refractory to other treatments.

- **Multidisciplinary Approach:** Physical therapy, psychological support, and pain management for chronic pelvic pain.

Complications:

- Chronic Pain: Leading to reduced quality of life.
- Infertility: Particularly in cases of untreated endometriosis or PID.
- Psychological Impact: Anxiety, depression, and sexual dysfunction.

Mcq 1: Which Of The Following Is The Most Likely Diagnosis For A Woman Presenting With Cyclic Pelvic Pain, Dysmenorrhea, And Dyspareunia?

- A) Ovarian Torsion
- B) Endometriosis
- C) Interstitial Cystitis
- D) Pelvic Inflammatory Disease

Answer: B) Endometriosis

Explanation: The symptoms of cyclic pelvic pain, dysmenorrhea, and dyspareunia are characteristic of endometriosis.

Mcq 2: What Is The First-Line Imaging Modality For Evaluating Acute Pelvic Pain In Women?

- A) MRI
- B) CT Scan
- C) Laparoscopy
- D) Pelvic Ultrasound

Answer: D) Pelvic Ultrasound

Explanation: Pelvic ultrasound is the first-line imaging modality for evaluating acute pelvic pain due to its accessibility, non-invasiveness, and ability to assess gynecological structures.

Clinical Scenario 1: A 28-year-old woman presents to the emergency department with sudden-onset severe right lower quadrant pain. She is nauseated and has had one episode of vomiting. On examination, she is tender in the right lower quadrant with guarding. An ultrasound shows an enlarged, edematous right ovary with reduced blood flow.

What is the most likely diagnosis, and what is the next step in management?

Answer: The most likely diagnosis is ovarian torsion. The next step in management is urgent surgical intervention to untwist the ovary and restore blood flow, ideally through laparoscopy.

Explanation: The presentation of acute severe pelvic pain, nausea, and ultrasound findings of an enlarged ovary with reduced blood flow are classic for ovarian torsion, which is a surgical emergency.

ENDOMETRIAL CANCER

Introduction: *Endometrial cancer is the most common gynecological malignancy in developed countries. It primarily affects postmenopausal women and arises from the lining of the uterus, known as the endometrium. The most common subtype is endometrioid adenocarcinoma, which is often related to excess estrogen exposure. Early detection and treatment are associated with a good prognosis, but advanced disease can be more challenging to manage.*

Pathophysiology: Endometrial cancer typically develops due to prolonged exposure to unopposed estrogen, which can stimulate the endometrial lining to undergo hyperplasia and, ultimately, malignant transformation. Conditions associated with increased estrogen exposure include obesity, polycystic ovary syndrome (PCOS), hormone replacement therapy (HRT) without progesterone, and tamoxifen use. Genetic factors, such as Lynch syndrome, also increase the risk of developing endometrial cancer.

Clinical Presentation: The most common symptom of endometrial cancer is abnormal uterine bleeding, especially in postmenopausal women. Premenopausal women may present with irregular or heavy menstrual bleeding. Other symptoms can include pelvic pain, dyspareunia (painful intercourse), and, in advanced cases, systemic symptoms like weight loss and fatigue.

Diagnosis: The initial evaluation of suspected endometrial cancer typically includes a transvaginal ultrasound to assess endometrial thickness. An endometrial biopsy is the gold standard for diagnosis. If the biopsy confirms cancer, further imaging, such as a pelvic MRI or CT scan, may be needed to assess the extent of the disease and guide treatment planning.

Management: The mainstay of treatment for endometrial cancer is surgery, which usually involves a total hysterectomy with bilateral salpingo-oophorectomy (removal of the uterus, fallopian tubes, and ovaries). In early-stage disease, surgery alone may be curative. Advanced disease may require additional treatments such as radiation therapy, chemotherapy, or hormone therapy, depending on the tumor's characteristics and stage.

Prognosis: The prognosis for endometrial cancer is generally favorable, especially when diagnosed at an early stage. The 5-year survival rate for localized endometrial cancer is over 90%. However, survival rates decrease significantly with advanced disease or high-risk histological subtypes.

Clinical Scenarios

Scenario 1:
A 62-year-old woman presents with postmenopausal bleeding. She had her last menstrual period 12 years ago and has not experienced any vaginal bleeding since. Her medical history includes obesity and hypertension. She denies any pain or other symptoms.

Question : What is the most appropriate next step in the management of this patient?

Answer: The most appropriate next step is to perform a transvaginal ultrasound to assess the endometrial thickness.
Explanation: Postmenopausal bleeding is a red flag for

endometrial cancer. The first step in evaluating this patient is to measure the endometrial thickness using transvaginal ultrasound. If the endometrial thickness is greater than 4 mm, an endometrial biopsy should be performed to rule out malignancy. Given her risk factors, such as obesity, this patient is at an increased risk for endometrial cancer.

Scenario 2:
A 68-year-old woman with a history of early-stage endometrial cancer treated with a total hysterectomy 3 years ago presents for a routine follow-up. She reports no new symptoms and has been feeling well. Physical examination is unremarkable.

Question : What is the most appropriate follow-up for this patient at this stage?
Answer: The most appropriate follow-up for this patient includes regular physical examinations and possibly periodic imaging, depending on her initial cancer stage and grade.

Explanation: Follow-up care for patients treated for endometrial cancer typically involves regular physical exams to check for signs of recurrence, which most commonly occurs within the first 3 years after treatment. If she had a low-risk early-stage cancer, imaging might not be necessary unless there are symptoms suggestive of recurrence. However, for higher-risk cases, periodic imaging such as a pelvic ultrasound or CT scan might be recommended.

CERVICAL CANCER

Introduction: *Cervical cancer is the fourth most common cancer in women worldwide, and it primarily affects women in their reproductive years. It is a malignant neoplasm that originates in the cervix, the lower part of the uterus that connects to the vagina. The primary cause of cervical cancer is persistent infection with high-risk types of human papillomavirus (HPV), particularly HPV 16 and 18. Due to the introduction of screening programs and HPV vaccination, the incidence and mortality rates of cervical cancer have decreased significantly in developed countries.*

Pathophysiology: Cervical cancer typically develops through a series of precancerous changes known as cervical intraepithelial neoplasia (CIN), which is classified into three grades (CIN 1, 2, and 3) based on the extent of dysplasia. High-risk HPV types integrate into the host cell genome, leading to the production of viral oncoproteins E6 and E7. These oncoproteins inactivate tumor suppressor proteins p53 and Rb, resulting in uncontrolled cell proliferation and the eventual development of invasive cervical cancer.

Risk Factors: The primary risk factor for cervical cancer is persistent infection with high-risk HPV. Other risk factors include early onset of sexual activity, multiple sexual partners, a history of sexually transmitted infections, smoking, immunosuppression (e.g., HIV infection), long-term use of oral contraceptives, and low socioeconomic status.

Clinical Presentation: Cervical cancer often presents with abnormal vaginal bleeding, particularly postcoital bleeding, intermenstrual bleeding, or postmenopausal bleeding. Other symptoms may include vaginal discharge, pelvic pain, and, in advanced cases, symptoms related to local invasion such as urinary or bowel symptoms.

Diagnosis: The diagnosis of cervical cancer is typically made through a combination of cervical cytology (Pap smear), HPV testing, and colposcopy with biopsy. If invasive cancer is suspected, further evaluation with imaging studies such as MRI, CT scan, or PET-CT may be necessary to assess the extent of the disease and guide treatment planning.

Management: The management of cervical cancer depends on the stage of the disease. Early-stage disease (stage IA1 to IB1) is usually treated with surgical options, including conization, radical hysterectomy, or trachelectomy (for fertility preservation). More advanced stages may require a combination of radiation therapy and chemotherapy. The prognosis for cervical cancer is favorable if detected early, with a 5-year survival rate exceeding 90% for localized disease. However, the prognosis worsens with advanced stages.

Prevention: Primary prevention of cervical cancer is achieved through HPV vaccination, which is highly effective in preventing infection with the most common high-risk HPV types. Secondary prevention is accomplished through regular cervical cancer screening with Pap smears and HPV testing, which can detect precancerous lesions that can be treated before they progress to invasive cancer.

Clinical Scenarios

Scenario 1:
A 32-year-old woman presents for her annual gynecological examination. She reports no symptoms and has had regular Pap smears in the past. Her last Pap smear three years ago was normal.

She is not sexually active and has never received the HPV vaccine.

Question 1: What is the most appropriate screening recommendation for this patient?

Answer: The most appropriate screening recommendation is to perform a Pap smear combined with HPV testing (co-testing) at this visit.

Explanation: Current guidelines recommend that women aged 30-65 undergo cervical cancer screening with a Pap smear and HPV testing (co-testing) every 5 years, or a Pap smear alone every 3 years. Despite her previous normal Pap smear, co-testing is recommended due to her age, and the fact that she has not received the HPV vaccine. HPV testing is important as it can identify high-risk types of the virus that are associated with cervical cancer.

Scenario 2:
A 45-year-old woman presents with postcoital bleeding for the past two months. She has not had a Pap smear in over 10 years. On physical examination, the cervix appears friable with an irregular, exophytic mass.

Question 2: What is the next step in the management of this patient?

Answer: The next step is to perform a colposcopy with a directed biopsy of the cervical lesion.

Explanation: Postcoital bleeding, especially in the presence of a visible cervical mass, is highly suspicious for cervical cancer. The priority is to obtain a tissue diagnosis through colposcopy and biopsy. Colposcopy allows for the detailed examination of the cervix, and biopsies can confirm the presence of malignant cells. If cervical cancer is confirmed, further imaging will be necessary to stage the disease.

Scenario 3:
A 60-year-old woman with a history of stage IB2 cervical cancer treated with chemoradiation one year ago presents with pelvic pain and difficulty urinating. She also reports weight loss and fatigue. A pelvic examination reveals a fixed pelvic mass.

Question 3: What is the most likely cause of her symptoms, and what is the next appropriate step?

Answer: The most likely cause of her symptoms is a recurrence of cervical cancer. The next appropriate step is to perform imaging studies, such as an MRI or PET-CT, to assess the extent of the disease.

Explanation: The patient's symptoms of pelvic pain, difficulty urinating, and weight loss, combined with a history of cervical cancer, suggest a possible recurrence. Recurrent cervical cancer often presents with local symptoms due to tumor growth or invasion into adjacent structures. Imaging studies are essential to evaluate the extent of the recurrence and to determine the best course of treatment, which may include surgery, further radiation, or palliative care depending on the extent of the disease.

GYNECOLOGICAL SCREENING

Introduction: *Gynecological screening is a crucial aspect of women's health, aimed at detecting diseases early, before they cause symptoms or complications. The most common screenings in gynecology include cervical cancer screening (Pap smear and HPV testing), breast cancer screening (mammography), and screening for sexually transmitted infections (STIs). These screenings are guided by age, risk factors, and personal and family medical histories.*

Cervical Cancer Screening: Cervical cancer screening is primarily done through the Pap smear, which involves collecting cells from the cervix to detect precancerous changes or cancer. Human papillomavirus (HPV) testing can also be performed simultaneously. The introduction of the HPV vaccine has significantly reduced the incidence of cervical cancer, but screening remains essential, particularly for those who have not been vaccinated or who have a history of HPV infection.

• *Pap Smear:* Recommended every 3 years for women aged 21-29 and every 3-5 years for women aged 30-65 when combined with HPV testing (co-testing).
• *HPV Testing:* Often combined with the Pap smear for women aged 30 and older, as it helps identify those at high risk for cervical cancer.

Breast Cancer Screening: Breast cancer screening typically involves mammography, an X-ray of the breast used to detect early signs of breast cancer. Breast self-exams and clinical breast exams are also part of routine care, though their effectiveness as screening tools is debated.
• *Mammography:* Recommended annually or biennially for

women aged 40-74, depending on individual risk factors. Women at higher risk may start screening earlier and may need more frequent screenings or additional imaging, such as MRI.

Sexually Transmitted Infection (STI) Screening: Routine STI screening is vital for sexually active women, especially those under 25 or at increased risk (e.g., multiple sexual partners, history of STIs).
- *Chlamydia and Gonorrhea:* Recommended annually for sexually active women under 25 and for older women at increased risk.
- *HIV Screening:* Recommended for all sexually active women at least once, with more frequent testing for those at higher risk.
- *Other STIs:* Screening for syphilis, hepatitis B, and C may be indicated based on risk factors.

Other Screenings:
- **Osteoporosis:** Bone density screening with dual-energy X-ray absorptiometry (DEXA) is recommended for women aged 65 and older or younger women with risk factors for osteoporosis.
- **Ovarian Cancer:** Routine screening for ovarian cancer is not recommended for average-risk women due to the lack of effective screening tests. However, women with a strong family history may undergo genetic testing and possibly more frequent ultrasounds and CA-125 blood tests.

Clinical Scenarios

Scenario 1:
A 24-year-old sexually active woman presents for a routine check-up. She has no symptoms and has never had an STI. She reports having a new sexual partner in the past year and has not used condoms consistently.

Question 1: What screening tests should be performed during this visit?

Answer: The appropriate screening tests include a Pap smear (if not already done) and testing for chlamydia and gonorrhea.

Explanation: The patient is at increased risk for STIs due to her age and inconsistent condom use with a new sexual partner. Annual screening for chlamydia and gonorrhea is recommended for sexually active women under 25. A Pap smear is also recommended if she has not had one since turning 21, though HPV testing is not typically recommended until age 30 unless there are specific risk factors.

Scenario 2:
A 50-year-old woman with no significant medical history presents for a routine gynecological exam. Her last Pap smear was 3 years ago, and her last mammogram was 2 years ago. She is not sexually active and has no family history of breast or ovarian cancer.

Question 2: What are the recommended screenings for this patient?

Answer: The recommended screenings include a Pap smear with HPV testing (co-testing) and a mammogram.

Explanation: For a woman aged 50, it is recommended to perform a Pap smear with HPV testing every 5 years (or a Pap smear alone every 3 years). Additionally, mammography is recommended every 1-2 years for women aged 40-74. Despite the lack of symptoms or family history, regular screening is essential for early detection of cervical and breast cancers.

Scenario 3:

A 35-year-old woman with a strong family history of breast and ovarian cancer (her mother was diagnosed with breast cancer at age 40) presents for genetic counseling. She is concerned about her risk and asks about screening options.

Question 3: What screening recommendations should be made for this patient?

Answer: The patient should be offered genetic testing for BRCA1 and BRCA2 mutations, and depending on the results, she may need earlier and more frequent mammography or MRI screening, as well as consideration of risk-reducing options like prophylactic surgery.

Explanation: A strong family history of breast and ovarian cancer, especially with a first-degree relative diagnosed before age 50, warrants genetic counseling and testing for BRCA mutations. If she tests positive, enhanced surveillance with earlier and more frequent breast cancer screening, including MRI, may be recommended. Additionally, discussions about prophylactic mastectomy or oophorectomy may be appropriate depending on her risk profile and personal preferences.

MIXED Q&A

1. Which Of The Following Is The Most Common Cause Of Primary Amenorrhea?

- A) Turner syndrome
- B) Mayer-Rokitansky-Küster-Hauser syndrome
- C) Polycystic Ovary Syndrome (PCOS)
- D) Androgen Insensitivity Syndrome

Answer: A) Turner syndrome

Explanation: Turner syndrome, characterized by the presence of a single X chromosome (45,X), is the most common cause of primary amenorrhea. It is associated with ovarian dysgenesis and the absence of secondary sexual characteristics.

2. Which Of The Following Is The Most Appropriate Initial Management For A Patient With A Bartholin Cyst?

- A) Antibiotics
- B) Marsupialization
- C) Word catheter insertion
- D) Incision and drainage

Answer: C) Word catheter insertion

Explanation: Word catheter insertion is the preferred initial management for a symptomatic Bartholin cyst. It allows continuous drainage and facilitates healing. Marsupialization is considered if recurrent.

3. A 32-Year-Old Woman Presents With Irregular Menstrual Cycles And Hirsutism. Which Of The Following Is The Most Likely Diagnosis?

- A) Cushing syndrome
- B) Polycystic Ovary Syndrome (PCOS)
- C) Hyperprolactinemia
- D) Congenital adrenal hyperplasia

Answer: B) Polycystic Ovary Syndrome (PCOS)

Explanation: PCOS is the most common cause of irregular menstrual cycles and hirsutism in women of reproductive age. It is associated with hyperandrogenism and chronic anovulation.

4. Which Of The Following Is The Recommended Screening Test For Cervical Cancer?

- A) Pelvic ultrasound
- B) Colposcopy
- C) Pap smear
- D) HPV DNA test

Answer: C) Pap smear

Explanation: The Pap smear is the recommended screening test for cervical cancer. It detects precancerous and cancerous cells in the cervix. HPV DNA testing is also used but typically as an adjunct to or follow-up for abnormal Pap results.

5. Which Of The Following Is The Most Common Cause Of Postmenopausal Bleeding?

- A) Endometrial cancer
- B) Endometrial atrophy

- C) Endometrial hyperplasia
- D) Uterine fibroids

Answer: B) Endometrial atrophy

Explanation: Endometrial atrophy is the most common cause of postmenopausal bleeding. However, endometrial cancer must be ruled out in any postmenopausal woman presenting with bleeding.

6. A 28-Year-Old Woman Presents With Severe Dysmenorrhea And Pelvic Pain. Laparoscopy Reveals Endometriotic Lesions. What Is The First-Line Treatment?

- A) Oral contraceptives
- B) GnRH agonists
- C) Danazol
- D) NSAIDs

Answer: A) Oral contraceptives

Explanation: Oral contraceptives are often the first-line treatment for endometriosis-related pain. They work by suppressing ovulation and reducing menstrual flow, which can alleviate symptoms.

7. Which Of The Following Is The Most Common Type Of Ovarian Tumor In Women Under 30 Years Of Age?

- A) Serous cystadenoma
- B) Dermoid cyst (mature cystic teratoma)
- C) Endometrioma
- D) Mucinous cystadenoma

Answer: B) Dermoid cyst (mature cystic teratoma)

Explanation: Dermoid cysts, or mature cystic teratomas, are the most common type of ovarian tumor in women under 30 years of age. They are benign germ cell tumors.

8. Which Of The Following Is A Risk Factor For The Development Of Endometrial Cancer?

- A) Multiparity
- B) Use of oral contraceptives
- C) Obesity
- D) Early menopause

Answer: C) Obesity

Explanation: Obesity is a significant risk factor for endometrial cancer due to increased estrogen levels from peripheral conversion of androgens in adipose tissue.

9. A 25-Year-Old Nulliparous Woman Presents With A 6 Cm Ovarian Cyst. What Is The Most Appropriate Management?

- A) Immediate surgery
- B) Serial ultrasound monitoring
- C) Oral contraceptive pills
- D) Aspiration of the cyst

Answer: B) Serial ultrasound monitoring

Explanation: For a simple ovarian cyst in a young, asymptomatic woman, serial ultrasound monitoring is appropriate. Most cysts resolve spontaneously. Surgery is reserved for cysts that persist or have concerning features.

10. Which Of The Following Is The Most

Appropriate Next Step In The Management Of A Postmenopausal Woman With An Endometrial Thickness Of 8 Mm On Ultrasound?

- A) Reassurance and follow-up
- B) Endometrial biopsy
- C) Hormone replacement therapy
- D) Hysterectomy

Answer: B) Endometrial biopsy

Explanation: An endometrial thickness greater than 4 mm in a postmenopausal woman warrants further evaluation, typically with an endometrial biopsy, to rule out endometrial cancer.
Matching Questions

11. Match The Following Conditions With Their Most Common Associated Symptom:

- A) Endometriosis
- B) Polycystic Ovary Syndrome (PCOS)
- C) Pelvic Inflammatory Disease (PID)
- D) Ectopic Pregnancy

e. Irregular menstrual cycles
f. Pelvic pain
g. Severe lower abdominal pain with adnexal tenderness
h. Shoulder pain

Answers:

- A) Endometriosis - f) Pelvic pain
- B) Polycystic Ovary Syndrome (PCOS) - e) Irregular menstrual cycles
- C) Pelvic Inflammatory Disease (PID) - g) Severe lower abdominal pain with adnexal tenderness

- o   D) Ectopic Pregnancy - h) Shoulder pain

Explanation:
- o   Endometriosis is often associated with chronic pelvic pain.
- o   PCOS is commonly associated with irregular menstrual cycles due to anovulation.
- o   PID presents with severe lower abdominal pain, often with adnexal tenderness.
- o   Ectopic pregnancy can cause shoulder pain due to diaphragmatic irritation from blood in the peritoneal cavity.

12. Match The Following Gynecological Malignancies With Their Most Common Risk Factor:

- o   A) Cervical cancer
- o   B) Ovarian cancer
- o   C) Endometrial cancer
- o   D) Vaginal cancer

- e.   Human papillomavirus (HPV) infection
- f.   Family history of BRCA mutations
- g.   Unopposed estrogen exposure
- h.   Diethylstilbestrol (DES) exposure

Answers:
- o   A) Cervical cancer - e) Human papillomavirus (HPV) infection
- o   B) Ovarian cancer - f) Family history of BRCA mutations
- o   C) Endometrial cancer - g) Unopposed estrogen exposure
- o   D) Vaginal cancer - h) Diethylstilbestrol (DES) exposure

Explanation:
- o   HPV infection is the primary cause of cervical cancer.

- BRCA mutations significantly increase the risk of ovarian cancer.
- Unopposed estrogen exposure, such as in obesity or hormone replacement therapy without progesterone, increases the risk of endometrial cancer.
- DES exposure in utero is associated with an increased risk of clear cell adenocarcinoma of the vagina.

Direct Questions

13. What Is The First-Line Antibiotic Therapy For Treating Pelvic Inflammatory Disease (Pid)?

Answer: Ceftriaxone plus doxycycline with or without metronidazole

Explanation: The first-line treatment for PID typically includes a combination of antibiotics to cover the likely pathogens, which include Neisseria gonorrhoeae, Chlamydia trachomatis, and anaerobic bacteria.

14. What Is The Definitive Treatment For Severe Uterine Prolapse?

Answer: Hysterectomy with pelvic floor repair

Explanation: Hysterectomy with pelvic floor repair is the definitive treatment for severe uterine prolapse, particularly in women who do not desire future fertility.

15. What Is The Most Common Side Effect Of Long-Term Tamoxifen Therapy In Postmenopausal Women?

Answer: Endometrial hyperplasia or cancer

Explanation: Tamoxifen, a selective estrogen receptor modulator, has an estrogenic effect on the endometrium, increasing the risk of endometrial hyperplasia and cancer in postmenopausal women.

16. What Is The Most Appropriate Initial Test To Evaluate An Adnexal Mass In A Premenopausal Woman?

Answer: Pelvic ultrasound

Explanation: Pelvic ultrasound is the initial imaging modality of choice for evaluating adnexal masses, providing information about the size, location, and characteristics of the mass.

17. What Is The Primary Indication For Performing A Colposcopy?

Answer: Abnormal Pap smear results

Explanation: Colposcopy is performed when a Pap smear indicates the presence of atypical or abnormal cells, to further evaluate the cervix and obtain directed biopsies.

18. What Is The Preferred Method Of Contraception For A Breastfeeding Woman?

Answer: Progestin-only contraceptives (e.g., progestin-only pill, IUD, or implant)

Explanation: Progestin-only contraceptives are preferred in breastfeeding women as they do not affect milk production and have a low risk of side effects for the infant.

19. Which Hormone Is Primarily Responsible For Ovulation?

Answer: Luteinizing hormone (LH)

Explanation: The surge in luteinizing hormone (LH) triggers ovulation, releasing the mature oocyte from the follicle.

20. What Is The Gold Standard For Diagnosing Endometriosis?

Answer: Laparoscopy with biopsy

Explanation: Laparoscopy with biopsy is the gold standard for diagnosing endometriosis, allowing direct visualization and histological confirmation of endometrial tissue outside the uterus.

21. What Is The Most Common Complication Of A Hysterosalpingogram?

Answer: Pelvic infection

Explanation: The most common complication of a hysterosalpingogram, a radiologic procedure used to evaluate the fallopian tubes and uterine cavity, is pelvic infection, particularly in the presence of a preexisting tubal infection.

22. What Is The Most Appropriate Treatment For A Hemodynamically Stable Patient With A Ruptured Ectopic Pregnancy?

Answer: Laparoscopic salpingectomy

Explanation: Laparoscopic salpingectomy is the treatment of choice for a ruptured ectopic pregnancy in a hemodynamically stable patient. It involves removing the affected fallopian tube.

23. Describe The Pathophysiology Of Polycystic Ovary Syndrome (Pcos).

Answer: PCOS is characterized by hyperandrogenism, chronic anovulation, and polycystic ovaries. It is often associated with insulin resistance, leading to an increase in insulin levels that further stimulate androgen production by the ovaries. This results in the suppression of normal follicular development, causing anovulation and menstrual irregularities.

24. What Is The Role Of Gnrh Agonists In The Management Of Fibroids?

Answer: GnRH agonists, such as leuprolide, reduce estrogen levels by downregulating GnRH receptors in the pituitary gland, leading to a temporary menopausal state. This results in a reduction in fibroid size and symptomatic relief, often used as a preoperative treatment.

25. Explain The Mechanism Of Action Of Oral Contraceptives In Preventing Pregnancy.

Answer: Oral contraceptives typically contain estrogen and progestin, which prevent pregnancy by inhibiting ovulation, thickening cervical mucus to block sperm entry, and altering the endometrium to prevent implantation.

26. What Is The Significance Of An Elevated Ca-125 Level In A Postmenopausal Woman?

Answer: An elevated CA-125 level in a postmenopausal woman may indicate the presence of ovarian cancer, although it is not specific and can be elevated in other conditions like endometriosis, pelvic inflammatory disease, and benign ovarian cysts. It is often used in conjunction with imaging and clinical findings to guide further investigation.

27. How Does Tamoxifen Increase The Risk Of Endometrial Cancer?

Answer: Tamoxifen acts as an estrogen agonist in the endometrium, promoting endometrial proliferation, which can lead to hyperplasia and increase the risk of endometrial cancer. This is particularly a concern in postmenopausal women.

28. What Are The Indications For Performing A Cesarean Section?

Answer: Indications for cesarean section include fetal distress, abnormal fetal lie (e.g., breech or transverse), placental abruption, placenta previa, failed labor progression, uterine rupture, and maternal conditions such as severe preeclampsia or eclampsia.

29. What Are The Criteria For Diagnosing Preeclampsia?

Answer: Preeclampsia is diagnosed based on the presence of hypertension (≥140/90 mmHg) after 20 weeks of gestation, accompanied by proteinuria (≥300 mg/24 hours) or evidence of end-organ dysfunction (e.g., thrombocytopenia, elevated liver enzymes, renal insufficiency, pulmonary edema, or cerebral/visual symptoms).

30. What Is The Role Of Methotrexate In The Treatment Of Ectopic Pregnancy?

Answer: Methotrexate is used as a medical treatment for early, unruptured ectopic pregnancies. It inhibits cell division by interfering with DNA synthesis, thus allowing the body to absorb the ectopic tissue without the need for surgery.

Multiple-Choice Questions (MCQs)

31. Which Of The Following Is The Most Common Symptom Of Uterine Fibroids?

- o A) Pelvic pain
- o B) Heavy menstrual bleeding
- o C) Infertility
- o D) Urinary frequency

Answer: B) Heavy menstrual bleeding

Explanation: The most common symptom of uterine fibroids (leiomyomas) is heavy menstrual bleeding, also known as menorrhagia. This can lead to anemia if untreated.

32. Which Of The Following Medications Is Most Appropriate For Treating Severe Menopausal Symptoms In A Woman With An Intact Uterus?

- o A) Estrogen-only therapy
- o B) Progestin-only therapy
- o C) Combined estrogen and progestin therapy
- o D) Selective serotonin reuptake inhibitor (SSRI)

Answer: C) Combined estrogen and progestin therapy

Explanation: In women with an intact uterus, combined estrogen and progestin therapy is recommended to prevent endometrial hyperplasia and cancer, which can be induced by unopposed estrogen.

33. Which Of The Following Is The Most Common Cause Of Infertility In Women?

- A) Endometriosis
- B) Polycystic Ovary Syndrome (PCOS)
- C) Tubal factor infertility
- D) Uterine abnormalities

Answer: B) Polycystic Ovary Syndrome (PCOS)

Explanation: PCOS is the most common cause of infertility in women, primarily due to chronic anovulation. It is characterized by hyperandrogenism and multiple ovarian cysts.

34. What Is The Most Appropriate Treatment For A Pregnant Woman Diagnosed With Asymptomatic Bacteriuria?

- A) Nitrofurantoin
- B) Trimethoprim-sulfamethoxazole
- C) Ciprofloxacin
- D) Doxycycline

Answer: A) Nitrofurantoin

Explanation: Nitrofurantoin is a safe and effective antibiotic for treating asymptomatic bacteriuria in pregnancy. It is preferred due to its safety profile and efficacy against common uropathogens.

35. Which Of The Following Conditions Is Most Commonly Associated With A Molar Pregnancy?

- A) Hyperemesis gravidarum
- B) Severe hypertension
- C) Hyperthyroidism
- D) Diabetes mellitus

Answer: A) Hyperemesis gravidarum

Explanation: Molar pregnancy, or hydatidiform mole, is often associated with excessive nausea and vomiting (hyperemesis gravidarum) due to high levels of hCG, which is produced by the trophoblastic tissue.

36. Which Of The Following Is The Most Appropriate Management For A 20-Year-Old Woman With A Simple Ovarian Cyst Measuring 4 Cm?

- A) Immediate surgical removal
- B) Repeat ultrasound in 6-12 weeks
- C) Oral contraceptive pills
- D) MRI of the pelvis

Answer: B) Repeat ultrasound in 6-12 weeks

Explanation: A simple ovarian cyst less than 5 cm in a young woman is usually benign and often resolves on its own. Repeat ultrasound in 6-12 weeks is appropriate to monitor for resolution.

37. Which Of The Following Is A Contraindication To The Use Of Combined Oral Contraceptives?

- A) History of migraines with aura
- B) Iron-deficiency anemia
- C) Family history of breast cancer
- D) Age over 35 with no other risk factors

Answer: A) History of migraines with aura

Explanation: Combined oral contraceptives are contraindicated in women with a history of migraines with aura due to an increased risk of stroke.

38. Which Of The Following Is The Most Common Presenting Symptom Of Endometrial Cancer?

- A) Postmenopausal bleeding
- B) Pelvic pain
- C) Weight loss
- D) Urinary incontinence

Answer: A) Postmenopausal bleeding

Explanation: Postmenopausal bleeding is the most common presenting symptom of endometrial cancer. Any postmenopausal bleeding warrants investigation to rule out malignancy.

39. What Is The Primary Treatment For Stage I Cervical Cancer?

- A) Chemotherapy
- B) Radiation therapy
- C) Radical hysterectomy
- D) Observation

Answer: C) Radical hysterectomy

Explanation: Radical hysterectomy is the primary treatment for stage I cervical cancer, especially in women who are not candidates for fertility preservation. It involves removal of the uterus, cervix, and surrounding tissues.

40. Which Of The Following Is A Characteristic Feature Of Lichen Sclerosus?

- A) Thin, white, wrinkled skin of the vulva
- B) Thickened, hyperpigmented skin of the vulva
- C) Papular lesions on the vulva
- D) Ulcerative lesions with yellow exudate

Answer: A) Thin, white, wrinkled skin of the vulva

Explanation: Lichen sclerosus is a chronic inflammatory condition that affects the vulvar skin, leading to thinning, whiteness, and a wrinkled appearance. It can cause significant discomfort and itching.

Matching Questions

41. Match The Following Gynecological Procedures With Their Primary Indication:

- A) LEEP (Loop Electrosurgical Excision Procedure)
- B) Dilation and Curettage (D&C)
- C) Endometrial ablation
- D) Tubal ligation

e. Treatment of cervical intraepithelial neoplasia
f. Endometrial sampling for abnormal uterine bleeding
g. Permanent contraception
h. Management of menorrhagia in women who have completed childbearing

Answers:

- A) LEEP - e) Treatment of cervical intraepithelial neoplasia
- B) Dilation and Curettage (D&C) - f) Endometrial sampling for abnormal uterine bleeding
- C) Endometrial ablation - h) Management of menorrhagia in women who have completed childbearing
- D) Tubal ligation - g) Permanent contraception

Explanation:

- LEEP is used to treat cervical intraepithelial neoplasia by excising abnormal tissue.

- o D&C is often performed to obtain endometrial samples in cases of abnormal uterine bleeding.
- o Endometrial ablation is a treatment for menorrhagia, reducing menstrual flow in women who no longer desire fertility.
- o Tubal ligation is a form of permanent contraception.

42. Match The Following Ovarian Cyst Types With Their Common Characteristics:

- o A) Dermoid cyst (Mature cystic teratoma)
- o B) Endometrioma
- o C) Follicular cyst
- o D) Theca lutein cyst

u. Contains elements from all three germ layers
v. Often associated with endometriosis
w. Result of failure of follicle rupture
x. Associated with high levels of hCG

Answers:

- o A) Dermoid cyst (Mature cystic teratoma) - u) Contains elements from all three germ layers
- o B) Endometrioma - v) Often associated with endometriosis
- o C) Follicular cyst - w) Result of failure of follicle rupture
- o D) Theca lutein cyst - x) Associated with high levels of hCG

Explanation:
- o Dermoid cysts (mature cystic teratomas) are composed of tissues from all three germ layers.
- o Endometriomas, or "chocolate cysts," are associated with endometriosis and contain old blood.
- o Follicular cysts occur when a dominant follicle fails to rupture and release an egg.
- o Theca lutein cysts are associated with high hCG levels, often seen in molar pregnancies or multiple gestations.

43. What Is The Primary Mechanism Of Action Of Gnrh Agonists In Treating Endometriosis?

Answer: GnRH agonists suppress the production of estrogen by downregulating GnRH receptors in the pituitary gland, leading to a hypoestrogenic state. This reduces the stimulation of endometriotic implants and helps alleviate pain and other symptoms associated with endometriosis.

44. Explain The Significance Of An Elevated Afp (Alpha-Fetoprotein) Level In A Pregnant Woman.

Answer: An elevated AFP level in pregnancy can indicate several conditions, including neural tube defects (e.g., spina bifida), abdominal wall defects (e.g., omphalocele), and multiple gestations. It may also be elevated in cases of incorrect dating of the pregnancy. Further evaluation with ultrasound and amniocentesis may be warranted.

45. What Is The Most Appropriate Management For A Pregnant Woman With Placenta Previa Diagnosed In The Third Trimester?

Answer: The management of placenta previa depends on the severity of bleeding and gestational age. If there is no active bleeding, the patient may be managed expectantly with close monitoring. If bleeding occurs, hospitalization and delivery via cesarean section at around 36-37 weeks are typically recommended to avoid maternal and fetal complications.

46. Describe The Pathophysiology Of Gestational Diabetes Mellitus (Gdm).

Answer: Gestational diabetes mellitus occurs when insulin resistance increases during pregnancy, often due to placental hormones like human placental lactogen (hPL). This insulin resistance leads to elevated blood glucose levels, which can affect both maternal and fetal health. GDM is typically diagnosed in the second or third trimester.

47. What Are The Potential Complications Of Untreated Pelvic Inflammatory Disease (Pid)?

Answer: Untreated pelvic inflammatory disease can lead to several complications, including chronic pelvic pain, infertility due to tubal scarring, ectopic pregnancy, and tubo-ovarian abscess. Prompt treatment with antibiotics is crucial to prevent these complications.

48. Explain The Clinical Significance Of A "Snowstorm" Appearance On Ultrasound In Early Pregnancy.

Answer: A "snowstorm" appearance on ultrasound is characteristic of a molar pregnancy (hydatidiform mole). This finding is due to the presence of numerous small cystic structures within the uterus, representing swollen chorionic villi. This condition requires prompt evacuation of the uterine contents and follow-up to monitor hCG levels.

49. What Are The Main Risk Factors For The Development Of Ovarian Cancer?

Answer: The main risk factors for ovarian cancer include advanced age, family history of ovarian or breast cancer, BRCA1 or BRCA2 gene mutations, nulliparity, early menarche, late menopause, and infertility. Use of oral contraceptives and multiparity are protective factors.

50. What Is The Role Of Bisphosphonates In The Management Of Postmenopausal Osteoporosis?

Answer: Bisphosphonates are used in the management of postmenopausal osteoporosis to reduce the risk of fractures. They work by inhibiting osteoclast-mediated bone resorption, thereby increasing bone mineral density. They are typically prescribed to women with a history of fractures or significant risk factors for osteoporosis.

Multiple-Choice Questions (Mcqs)

51. Which Of The Following Is The Best Initial Test For A Woman Presenting With Postmenopausal Bleeding?

- A) Pap smear
- B) Transvaginal ultrasound
- C) Endometrial biopsy
- D) Hysteroscopy

Answer: B) Transvaginal ultrasound

Explanation: Transvaginal ultrasound is the initial test of choice for evaluating postmenopausal bleeding as it measures endometrial thickness. If the endometrium is thicker than 4 mm, further evaluation with an endometrial biopsy may be needed.

52. What Is The Most Appropriate Next Step In The Management Of A Premenopausal Woman With A 3 Cm Asymptomatic Fibroadenoma?

- A) Immediate surgical excision
- B) Fine-needle aspiration
- C) Core needle biopsy
- D) Observation and follow-up ultrasound in 6 months

Answer: D) Observation and follow-up ultrasound in 6 months

Explanation: Asymptomatic fibroadenomas, especially those under 5 cm, can often be managed conservatively with observation and follow-up imaging to monitor for changes in size or characteristics.

53.Which Of The Following Is A Contraindication To Hormone Replacement Therapy (Hrt) In Postmenopausal Women?

- A) Severe vasomotor symptoms
- B) History of venous thromboembolism
- C) Osteoporosis
- D) Early menopause

Answer: B) History of venous thromboembolism

Explanation: Hormone replacement therapy is contraindicated in women with a history of venous thromboembolism due to an increased risk of clot formation associated with estrogen use.

54.Which Of The Following Is Most Indicative Of Bacterial Vaginosis?

- A) Thick, white, curd-like discharge
- B) Frothy, yellow-green discharge
- C) Thin, gray discharge with a fishy odor
- D) Purulent, yellow discharge with cervical motion tenderness

Answer: C) Thin, gray discharge with a fishy odor

Explanation: Bacterial vaginosis is characterized by a thin, gray discharge with a fishy odor, often due to the presence of anaerobic bacteria like Gardnerella vaginalis.

55.Which Of The Following Is A Risk Factor For

Developing Cervical Cancer?

- o   A) Multiparity
- o   B) Early age at first sexual intercourse
- o   C) Use of oral contraceptives
- o   D) Late menopause

Answer: B) Early age at first sexual intercourse

Explanation: Early sexual activity is a significant risk factor for cervical cancer, as it increases the likelihood of persistent human papillomavirus (HPV) infection, which is the primary cause of cervical cancer.

56. Which Type Of Ovarian Tumor Is Most Commonly Associated With Meigs Syndrome?

- o   A) Serous cystadenoma
- o   B) Mucinous cystadenoma
- o   C) Fibroma
- o   D) Dysgerminoma

Answer: C) Fibroma

Explanation: Meigs syndrome is a triad of ovarian fibroma, ascites, and pleural effusion. The condition typically resolves after the removal of the fibroma.

57. Which Of The Following Is The Most Common Cause Of Secondary Amenorrhea In Reproductive-Aged Women?

- o   A) Polycystic Ovary Syndrome (PCOS)
- o   B) Hyperprolactinemia
- o   C) Thyroid dysfunction
- o   D) Pregnancy

Answer: D) Pregnancy

Explanation: Pregnancy is the most common cause of secondary amenorrhea in women of reproductive age and should always be ruled out first with a pregnancy test.

58. What Is The Preferred Method For Screening For Gestational Diabetes Mellitus (Gdm)?

- A) Fasting plasma glucose
- B) 75-g Oral Glucose Tolerance Test (OGTT)
- C) Hemoglobin A1c
- D) Random blood glucose test

Answer: B) 75-g Oral Glucose Tolerance Test (OGTT)

Explanation: The 75-g OGTT is the preferred method for screening for gestational diabetes, typically performed between 24 and 28 weeks of gestation.

59. What Is The First-Line Treatment For Severe Preeclampsia At 35 Weeks Of Gestation?

- A) Bed rest and observation
- B) Administration of magnesium sulfate and induction of labor
- C) Oral antihypertensives and outpatient monitoring
- D) Cesarean section

Answer: B) Administration of magnesium sulfate and induction of labor

Explanation: Severe preeclampsia requires immediate management to prevent complications. Magnesium sulfate is given to prevent seizures, and induction of labor is initiated to deliver the fetus, as the definitive treatment for preeclampsia is delivery.

Matching Questions

60. Match The Following Hormonal Abnormalities With Their Associated Gynecological Conditions:

- A) Elevated androgen levels
- B) Elevated prolactin levels
- C) Decreased estrogen levels
- D) Elevated hCG levels

e. Polycystic Ovary Syndrome (PCOS)
f. Hyperprolactinemia
g. Menopause
h. Molar pregnancy

Answers:

- A) Elevated androgen levels - e) Polycystic Ovary Syndrome (PCOS)
- B) Elevated prolactin levels - f) Hyperprolactinemia
- C) Decreased estrogen levels - g) Menopause
- D) Elevated hCG levels - h) Molar pregnancy

Explanation:
- PCOS is characterized by elevated androgen levels leading to symptoms like hirsutism and acne.
- Hyperprolactinemia can cause amenorrhea and galactorrhea due to elevated prolactin levels.
- Menopause is associated with decreased estrogen levels, leading to symptoms like hot flashes and vaginal atrophy.
- Molar pregnancy produces excessively high levels of hCG, leading to symptoms such as severe nausea and hyperemesis

gravidarum.

61. Match The Following Gynecological Cancers With Their Most Common Histological Subtype:

- A) Ovarian cancer
- B) Endometrial cancer
- C) Cervical cancer
- D) Vulvar cancer

u. Serous adenocarcinoma
v. Endometrioid adenocarcinoma
w. Squamous cell carcinoma
x. Clear cell carcinoma

Answers:

- A) Ovarian cancer - u) Serous adenocarcinoma
- B) Endometrial cancer - v) Endometrioid adenocarcinoma
- C) Cervical cancer - w) Squamous cell carcinoma
- D) Vulvar cancer - w) Squamous cell carcinoma

Explanation:
- Serous adenocarcinoma is the most common subtype of epithelial ovarian cancer.
- Endometrioid adenocarcinoma is the most common type of endometrial cancer.
- Squamous cell carcinoma is the predominant histological subtype of cervical cancer, associated with HPV infection, and vulvar cancer.

Short-Answer Questions

62. Explain The Mechanism By Which Intrauterine Devices (Iuds) Prevent Pregnancy.

Answer: Intrauterine devices (IUDs) prevent pregnancy through different mechanisms depending on the type. Copper IUDs create an inflammatory response in the uterus, which is toxic to sperm and eggs, preventing fertilization. Hormonal IUDs release progestin, which thickens cervical mucus to prevent sperm from entering the uterus, thins the endometrial lining to prevent implantation, and may inhibit ovulation in some women.

63. What Is The Recommended Management For A Woman Diagnosed With Ovarian Torsion?

Answer: Ovarian torsion is a gynecological emergency that requires prompt surgical intervention. The recommended management is laparoscopic surgery to detorse the ovary and preserve ovarian function, if possible. If the ovary appears non-viable, oophorectomy may be necessary.

64. Describe The Stages Of Labor And The Key Events That Occur In Each Stage.

Answer:
o *Stage 1:* Begins with the onset of regular contractions and ends with full cervical dilation (10 cm). It is divided into the latent phase (slow cervical dilation) and the active phase (rapid cervical dilation).
o *Stage 2:* Begins with full cervical dilation and ends with the delivery of the baby. It involves the descent and expulsion of the fetus through the birth canal.
o *Stage 3:* Begins after the delivery of the baby and ends with the expulsion of the placenta. This stage involves the separation and delivery of the placenta.

65. What Is The Significance Of The "Triple Screen" Test In Pregnancy?

Answer: The "triple screen" test, typically performed between 15 and 20 weeks of gestation, measures levels of alpha-fetoprotein

(AFP), human chorionic gonadotropin (hCG), and estriol in maternal blood. It helps assess the risk of certain fetal conditions, including Down syndrome (trisomy 21), trisomy 18, and neural tube defects. Abnormal levels may warrant further testing, such as amniocentesis or detailed ultrasound.

66. What Are The Main Indications For Performing A Cesarean Section?

Answer: The main indications for cesarean section include fetal distress, abnormal fetal presentation (e.g., breech), placenta previa, uterine rupture, failure to progress in labor, maternal medical conditions (e.g., severe preeclampsia), and previous cesarean delivery (depending on the indication for the previous cesarean).

67. Explain The Physiological Changes That Occur In The Cardiovascular System During Pregnancy.

Answer: During pregnancy, the cardiovascular system undergoes several changes, including an increase in blood volume by 30-50%, a rise in cardiac output by 30-50%, a decrease in systemic vascular resistance, and a slight decrease in blood pressure during the second trimester. These changes accommodate the increased metabolic demands of the mother and fetus and improve placental blood flow.

68. What Is The Clinical Significance Of The "Chandelier Sign" In Gynecology?

Answer: The "Chandelier sign" refers to the extreme pain experienced by a patient during cervical motion tenderness, typically observed in pelvic inflammatory disease (PID). It indicates severe inflammation of the pelvic organs, often involving the uterus, fallopian tubes, and ovaries, and requires prompt antibiotic treatment.

69. What Is The Most Common Cause Of Abnormal Uterine Bleeding In Adolescent Females?

Answer: The most common cause of abnormal uterine bleeding in adolescent females is anovulation. During adolescence, the hypothalamic-pituitary-ovarian axis is often immature, leading to irregular cycles and anovulation, which results in unpredictable and heavy menstrual bleeding.

70. A 45-Year-Old Premenopausal Woman With A History Of Polycystic Ovary Syndrome (Pcos) Presents With Irregular Menstrual Cycles And Periods Of Heavy Bleeding Lasting For Several Weeks. She Has Not Been On Any Hormonal Therapy And Has A Bmi Of 35.

What is the most likely underlying pathophysiological mechanism contributing to her symptoms?

Answer: The most likely underlying mechanism is chronic anovulation leading to unopposed estrogen exposure.
Explanation: Women with PCOS often experience chronic anovulation, which results in unopposed estrogen exposure because they do not regularly ovulate and therefore do not produce progesterone, which counteracts estrogen. This can lead to endometrial hyperplasia and, over time, an increased risk of developing endometrial cancer. Her obesity further exacerbates this risk by contributing additional estrogen through peripheral conversion of androgens in adipose tissue.

71. A 28-Year-Old Woman Presents To The Clinic For A Routine Check-Up. She Has Been Sexually

Active With Multiple Partners In The Past But Has Been In A Monogamous Relationship For The Past Year. She Has Never Had A Pap Smear. She Reports No Symptoms But Is Concerned About Her Risk Of Cervical Cancer.

What is the recommended screening for this patient?

Answer: The recommended screening is a Pap smear.

Explanation: Cervical cancer screening should begin at age 21, regardless of sexual activity history. Since the patient is 28 and has never had a Pap smear, she should have one performed during this visit. If the Pap smear is normal, she should continue to have a Pap smear every 3 years. HPV testing is generally not recommended until age 30 unless there are specific risk factors. Since she has had multiple sexual partners in the past, it would also be prudent to consider STI screening, including tests for chlamydia and gonorrhea.

72: A 40-Year-Old Woman Presents For Her Annual Exam. She Has A Family History Of Cervical Cancer (Her Mother Was Diagnosed At Age 45) And Has Been Compliant With Regular Pap Smears, All Of Which Have Been Normal. She Is Concerned About Her Cancer Risk And Asks Whether She Should Have More Frequent Screening.

What is the appropriate advice regarding cervical cancer screening for this patient?

Answer: The patient should continue with regular screening according to guidelines, which means a Pap smear with HPV co-testing every 5 years or a Pap smear alone every 3 years.

Explanation: The patient's family history of cervical cancer (mother diagnosed at age 45) does not significantly alter the standard screening recommendations for cervical cancer, as most cases are related to HPV infection rather than a genetic predisposition. The current guidelines recommend co-testing (Pap smear plus HPV test) every 5 years or a Pap smear alone every 3 years for women aged 30-65 with a history of normal results. She does not need more frequent screening but should continue regular follow-up according to these guidelines. It is also important to discuss the role of HPV vaccination if she has not been vaccinated, although the primary benefit is in younger individuals before the onset of sexual activity.

ABOUT THE AUTHOR

Essam Abdelhakim

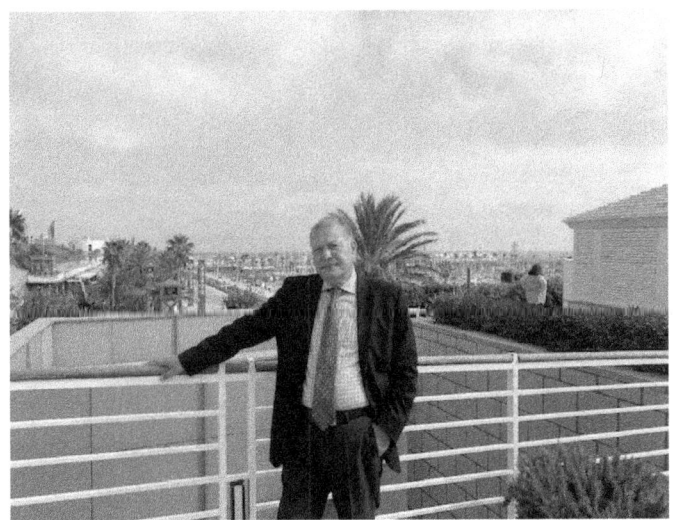

Senior consultant with Extensive Experience in Medical Education

DISCLOSURE

Disclosure

This book has been created with the assistance of *Artificial Intelligence (AI) tools* and thoroughly reviewed and edited by the author to ensure clarity, relevance, and educational value.

While every effort has been made to provide accurate and up-to-date information, this content is intended solely for educational and informational purposes.

The author is a medical professional; however, the information provided in this book *is not a substitute for professional medical advice, diagnosis, or treatment.*

Readers are strongly advised to consult licensed healthcare providers or specialists for any medical concerns or conditions.

By using this book, **you acknowledge and agree** that the author shall not be held responsible or liable for any loss, damage, or harm whether physical, emotional, financial, or otherwise that may occur *as a result of the use or misuse of the information presented herein.*

www.ingramcontent.com/pod-product-compliance
Lightning Source LLC
Chambersburg PA
CBHW071932210526
45479CB00002B/649